Praise for Jann Arden's Feeding My Mother

#1 NATIONAL BESTSELLER

"Arden discusses the grimmest moments of her life with a sense of humour so lively it's hard to smother a laugh even when the subject matter is painful." —THE GLOBE AND MAIL

"Honest, humorous and inspirational. . . . Immerse yourself in [Arden's] story and you'll be mesmerized and inspired by the sunny outlook she's known for." —CANADIAN LIVING

"Jann Arden is one of the most honest and talented women I've ever met, and her love for her mother is so rich." —CHEF LYNN CRAWFORD

"*Feeding My Mother* emphasizes the emotional power of cooking and feeding one another. The idea of relationship building and bonding over preparing and eating together is ever present." —EAT NORTH

"[*Feeding My Mother*] is a kind, sad and, in typical Arden fashion, funny look at a daughter becoming a parent to parents. It is a comfortable read that makes you feel like you are sitting at Arden's country kitchen table with a cup of tea in hand, listening while Arden and her mom talk about dog hair, old cats, pushy squirrels and what happened ten minutes ago." —VANCOUVER SUN

"Poignant." —TORONTO SUN

"[Arden] conveys the challenges of [her] situation while incorporating heartwarming highs." —BUSTLE

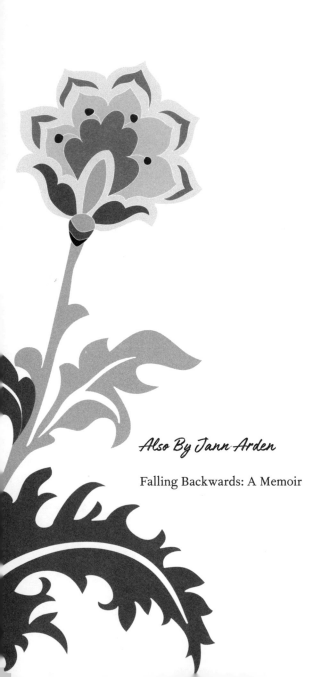

Also By Jann Arden

Falling Backwards: A Memoir

FEEDING MY MOTHER

Comfort and Laughter in the Kitchen as a
Daughter Lives with her Mom's Memory Loss

JANN ARDEN

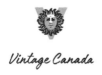

Vintage Canada

VINTAGE CANADA EDITION, 2019
Copyright © 2017 by Jann Arden

Published by Vintage Canada, a division of Penguin Random House Canada Limited, in 2019. Originally published in hardcover by Random House Canada, a division of Penguin Random House Canada Limited, in 2017. Distributed in Canada by Penguin Random House Canada Limited, Toronto.

Vintage Canada with colophon is a registered trademark.

www.penguinrandomhouse.ca

Library and Archives Canada Cataloguing in Publication

Arden, Jann, author
      Feeding my mother : comfort and laughter in the kitchen
as a daughter lives with her mom's memory loss / Jann Arden.

Previously published: Toronto: Random House Canada, 2017.

ISBN 978-0-7352-7393-1
eBook ISBN 9780735273948

      1. Arden, Jann—Family. 2. Alzheimer's disease—Patients—Care—Alberta.
3. Alzheimer's disease—Patients—Family relationships—Alberta.
4. Mothers and daughters—Alberta. 5. Musicians—Canada—Biography.
6. Caregivers—Alberta—Biography. 7. Alzheimer's disease—Patients—
Alberta—Biography. I. Title.

RC523.2A73 2019   362.1968'3110092   C2017-902278-4

Book design: Terri Nimmo
Photography by Jann Arden. Photographs of Jann and her mom: (viii, 191) Nadine Beauchesne; (vi) Paul Brandt.
Illustrations: (cover, ii) Nataliia Kucherenko, (7, 8, 29, 44, 77, 88, 93, 101, 108, 133) Irtsya; (162, 189) lozas / all from Shutterstock.com.

Printed and bound in the United States of America

2 4 6 8 9 7 5 3 1

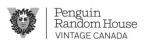

Penguin
Random House
VINTAGE CANADA

This book is dedicated with an abundance of love and gratitude
to my mom and dad, Joan and Derrel Richards.
Never judgmental.
Always understanding and supportive.
Forever facing forward.

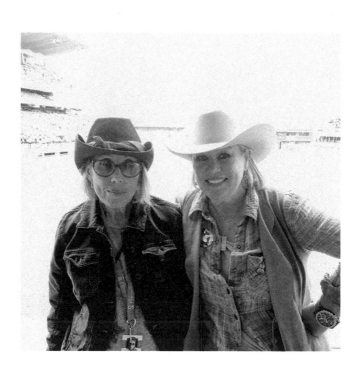

Another year, another page.
a million moments melt away.
The ticking-tocking hands of time,
what's found and lost, remains sublime.
The details that we hold so fast,
are nothing more than memories past.
For love is all that lingers true,
the bond that ties my heart to you.

—JANN ARDEN, DECEMBER 29, 2013

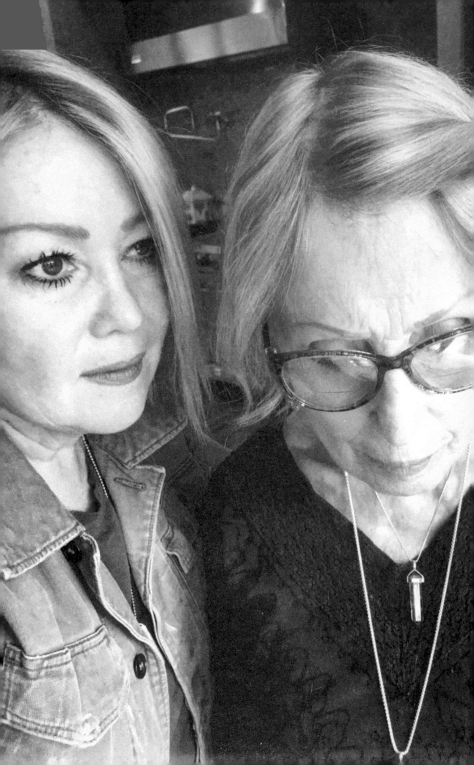

I remember the first day it happened.

I remember the first time she forgot something big. It wasn't the kind of lapse we all have from time to time—forgetting where we put our keys or our cell phones, or where we parked the car. This was a big sudden void. Right after it happened, that morning eight years ago now, I felt a discomfort insert itself at the back of my throat that hasn't really eased up since. It's hard for me to remember what my life used to feel like. It's hard for me to remember my old mom.

We had been sitting having a visit with my sister-in-law, Lori, talking about life things: the weather, the grandkids, jobs, the progress of our summer garden. Everything seemed perfectly normal. My sister-in-law at some point brought up the subject of her old cat. "I didn't want to tell you, Joan," she said to my mom, "but we had to have her put down a few days ago. God, whatever you guys do, don't tell Duray about it, as he'll be devastated."

My brother Duray was in jail, as he had been for the last twenty-five years, for first-degree murder—a murder he has always denied committing. He isn't really up to speed on what is going on around our lives out here in the free world, and he's very sensitive to anything the least bit upsetting. I'm sure it's because he feels so helpless. I think that's why Lori wanted to spare him the news about their cat.

"I would never say a word," Mom said. Lori went on about how sick the cat had been and that she hadn't found the right moment to tell Duray she was gone. We talked about it in detail for at least fifteen minutes. Mom seemed to be carefully listening to the story, consoling and responding in all the right places. Lori repeated again as she walked out the door, "Please don't say anything, okay, you guys?"

Mom said, "We won't, Lori. Mom's the word." And we all had a bit of a laugh.

Lori waved goodbye, hopped into her little blue compact and pulled out of the driveway.

Before the car had even disappeared down the road, Mom's phone rang, and it was Duray. The first thing that came out of her mouth, was, "You wouldn't believe it, but your cat died!" I stood there in her kitchen in disbelief.

"MOM!" I waved my arms in the air trying to get her attention.

"What?" she asked with her hand over the receiver. "I'm on the phone!"

"Jesus, you weren't supposed to tell him that!"

"Tell him what?" She looked at me blankly. She really didn't know what she wasn't supposed to tell him.

"About the cat dying! What are you thinking?"

That was the day. From one single second to the next, my life, my mom's life, my dad's life, my brothers' lives, the lives of all of our friends and family, were altered profoundly. My mom had started the journey down the lonely, confusing road called Alzheimer's disease.

I would spend the next two years in denial. I made excuses for both my parents over and over again as the memory thieves slowly stole things from right beneath our noses. I chalked the frequent lapses up to garden-variety old age and tried to leave it at that. My dad had had a stroke several years earlier, so we already knew he had severe memory and mobility issues, but my mom was the normal one. She was the glue that held everything together. She dedicated her days to looking after my dad, coordinating his appointments and doling out his medications. She looked after their house and their yard and their meals and all the driving. I desperately needed her to be okay and I was also too scared to think about what was happening.

I must have hoped if I ignored it enough, and wished it away often enough, my mom would start remembering again. But that's not the way Alzheimer's works. I have come to think of it as a cruel and haphazard sculptor. It chisels away at a person, one tiny piece at a time, exposing a mind to every form of loss and sadness. Uncovering every nerve and every bone and every vein. It doesn't stop until it cuts away the last breath. We lived through a small stretch in which my mom knew she was forgetting things.

It seemed only a matter of hours to me, but it was actually a short few months where she was aware of things going missing and time being lost and tasks being left undone. She admitted to me once or twice that she knew she was forgetting things. I will never forget her saying to me, "I know I can't remember the way I used to, Jann. It could always be worse, you know. I hope you never let me become a filthy old lady." Those words are stuck inside my heart like wet leaves in a gutter.

I have spent the last few years in various stages of grief and fear and frustration and anger. I'm not sure half the time if I am doing things right with my mom, or screwing things up, but I do know that none of that matters. What matters are the moments spent with the people you love. What matters is setting judgement and resentment aside so that tolerance and patience and kindness can move into your soul and live there in their forever home. Life is never dull. That's what Mom always says. "Life may be hard, but it's not dull. . . ."

Mom's journey, and my journey with her, is not over yet, and for that I am grateful. In these last nine years I have learned more about compassion and empathy and forgiveness than I ever thought possible. I've learned that something good can come from something bad: facing adversity can make you a much better version of yourself. I've learned that having a sense of humour is crucial in order to survive these trying days. I've also learned that feeding my mother, making her a great home-cooked meal, provides both of us with grace and solace and peace, that food is so important for our wellness and contentment. I don't cook for her anymore, since she's had to leave home for a place that can take care of all her needs, but at the end of the book I've included some of the recipes I dreamed up to tempt her. You can soothe pretty much any heartache with a loaf of bread and a hot bowl of soup!

And I've learned that writing it all down can save me, which is what I started doing when everything around me began to feel unsteady. Seeing what was happening in front of me on the page made it much less daunting. And sharing my thoughts and feelings on social media made all the difference. I guess I wanted to reach out and tell somebody, anybody, about what was happening to my family. I didn't want to feel alone in a room with Alzheimer's. I wanted to throw open every door and window and let the light in. I wanted to unload some of the burden of carrying my parents' secrets. I wanted to rid myself of this weird shame I was feeling because they were forgetting themselves. I started feeling like I was being forgotten too, lost in this pile of nothingness. It all seemed like such a mess, and some days it still does. Some days now it's so sad I can barely breathe. I was talking with a friend about how I was feeling a while ago, and she described how she felt orphaned when she lost her parents even though she was a grown-up. I think that's exactly how I feel, even though Mom is still here physically. I feel like an orphan.

It turned out that sending out an account of my daily adventures with my folks was life-changing. People started writing back, sharing their doubts and fears and frustrations with me. It changed everything in such a positive, wonderful way. I am so grateful to all of them—to all of you. It takes bravery to share your troubles. It takes grit and guts and gumption. Thank you for easing my troubles, for putting your wisdom and pain out there for everyone to benefit from. I can't tell you how many hours I've spent propped up in my bed reading through the hundreds and hundreds of comments you've left on my Facebook pages. I've laughed out loud and cried quietly and I have to say, I feel much less alone for having reached out. Losing someone an inch at a time is extremely hard.

—

This book is a glimpse into my journey with memory loss but it's also a journey that thousands and thousands of us are on with our mothers and fathers and sisters and brothers and husbands and wives and uncles and aunts and grandmothers and grandfathers and even children.

Alzheimer's and dementia have always been there, but perhaps families in earlier generations absorbed their elderly folks into the fold of home more gracefully. Many of us these days don't have the kind of lives or rooted family structures that enable us to cope with parents or grandparents who can't manage on their own, and we have to find nursing homes for them. Some of these places are great, some not so good, some downright depressing and dehumanizing. It's an agonizing decision and one that can be hard to live with. For a long time I was lucky enough to have the means to keep Mom at home with me, and find ways to meet the challenges that entails. The stories and the recipes in this book are what I have to share about how we're managing—about the road my mom and all the people who love her are travelling. It was written with humility, and sadness, and fear, and panic, and joy.

What I've learned is that no matter what comes you've got to wrap yourself in all the goodness you can muster. That's what my mom does every single day.

I remember once, when she was deep in the grip of dementia but still able to live at home, we were driving into town to buy a few groceries, she told me that she was eighty per cent happy. That made me laugh really hard. "Eighty per cent, Mom? Well, that's way better than me!"

She told me that I would have to work on that. . . .

Mom's journey, and my journey with her, is far from over and for that I am grateful.

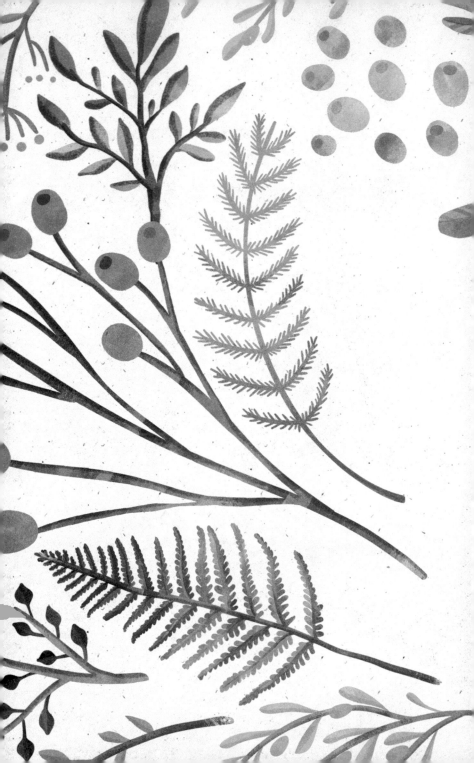

June 14, 2014

It's been an interesting, daunting, scary, anxiety-ridden week. Last Wednesday I ended up calling an ambulance to come and gather up my very delusional, incontinent, falling-all-over-the-place father. My mom and I had tried to "work through" whatever issues he was having for about forty-eight hours when I finally realized that it was something more than him just not feeling good. He couldn't answer my questions, and when he did try to answer, his responses were so abstract and zany we couldn't help but smile (through our fear).

It's difficult watching your parents getting older, and frailer, and increasingly more forgetful. I have watched some of my friends go through similar things with their folks over the past few years, and it's been agonizing to see them with such heavy hearts, so uncertain about what to do next. It's like one moment you are asking for permission to go to a high school dance and the next you're driving into town on a Depends run for your father.

It turns out my dad had some sort of "mystery infection" that triggered the apparent delirium. It's been squashed with antibiotics, but the doctor told us it can take months for an elderly person's mind to clear after such an infection. He has also been diagnosed with dementia, which we more or less knew, as it has come up before in some of his testing. He also has type 2 diabetes and some kidney issues and really crappy circulation in his legs, which makes it hard for him to walk. Other than that, he is super-healthy.

What do we do next?

Well, we want to bring him home. We are just trying to sort out what his needs are going to be once he gets here. So far, I think Mom and I will need:

- ✓ a Sherpa to get him up the stairs to his bedroom
- ✓ a comedian
- ✓ an award-winning food network chef
- ✓ a full-time housekeeper
- ✓ a butler
- ✓ a chauffeur
- ✓ a pharmacist
- ✓ a team of nurses
- ✓ a large oxygen tank
- ✓ one of those electric hospital beds
- ✓ a soft-serve ice cream machine
- ✓ a gardener
- ✓ and a drug dealer for my mother and myself.

Apparently the government will provide us with three hours a week of in-home help of some sort for free. What a load off our shoulders.

Seriously, though, you have to enter this stage of life with a sense of humour. Not only for your aging parents' sakes, but for yourself. Laughter is an amazing love potion and medicine—an incredible healer—and sometimes it's the help you need at the end of a long, hard, delirium-filled day.

June 15, 2014

My dad called Mom this morning from the hospital and asked her how *she* was. I thought that was adorable. I just need to secure the Sherpa and ice-cream machine and we can bring him home.

Well, my dad gets to come home today. Apparently he is already dressed and sitting on the edge of his bed, ready for us to pick him up.

Every time I went to visit him, he was lying in his bed with his brown leather shoes on. He told me that he was keeping them on his feet because things go missing around there. It made me laugh.

Life is funny. The subject of death can be, too. One day my mom told me that if Dad were to die in the yard, she and I would have to somehow get him into the wheelbarrow and push him up to the house so that the ambulance guys wouldn't have to do it. I am not kidding. Either that, she said, or we'd throw a tarp over him so the dogs wouldn't "get at him." Every time I look at the wheelbarrow now, I smile, thinking of my mom's way of solving problems.

She's never been sentimental. She looks at life with such economy and practicality. She lives in the day and doesn't get too far ahead of herself. When I was nine or ten, she told us at the supper table one night that we would all die one day and that we needed to try and have a happy life. That always stuck with me. To never talk about death is just plain silly. It's like not talking about one of the most important things in our existence.

I hope my dad has a happy summer. I hope he can sit in his lawn chair and yell at me about how I am using the weed eater wrong, or pruning the trees wrong, or hoeing the garden wrong. For some reason, I am looking forward to the old grouch hollering orders at me like I'm some waitress.

June 25, 2014

My dad has been home just over a week. He is so changed. His facial expressions, even his gestures, are somehow unfamiliar to

11

me—the way his mouth turns down at one corner, the way he looks past you over your shoulder, the way he holds his fork and knife like he is not sure what they're for. The grouchy, strict man who raised three kids, and poured concrete pads his whole life, has left the building. This man is quiet and still, perhaps wondering what his future holds. I catch him standing at the kitchen window looking down the road. His thumbs are shoved through his belt loops, and his jaw moves side to side.

You would think that my mother would be torn apart over losing (more or less) her partner of fifty-six years, but she's steady and calm and goes about her chores around the house without any visible sadness. She'll tell me, "Jann, that's just the way it goes. That's life. What can you do?" She never spends any time feeling sorry for herself—she has bird feeders to fill and squirrels to entertain, after all. She's tied strips of cloth— bits of cut-up tube socks and T-shirts and old aprons—to a dozen tree branches out in the yard. "The squirrels make their beds with them," she answered when I asked what in the hell they were for.

"That's weird, Mom."

"They love them. I put new ones out every few days because they all disappear."

She gets up in the morning and feeds the dogs and putters around. Makes herself and Dad a protein shake with anything that happens to be sitting on the kitchen counter, throwing bananas or nuts or apples into the blender with a scoop of "powder" as she calls it.

She vacuums every single day without fail and does at least one load of laundry. She never says, "I don't know what I'll do without your dad." She always tells me that she'll be fine, though she says she does worry sometimes. But that's what people do. They worry and let their brains run around like chickens in a slaughterhouse. That's what I do, too much of the time.

We are going to try and keep Dad at home. We'll make a few modifications in the bathrooms and we'll bubble-wrap everything. (Kidding.) That has always been the plan.

Mom and I think that Dad will outlive us. He always lands on his feet somehow, the guy who drank and smoked his whole life like some kind of movie star. He still has good days when he makes sense and bad days when we feel like we're playing charades as we try to figure out what he's trying to tell us.

Yesterday he called me and said, "I just wanted to touch base about your financial situation and whatnot." After many failed guesses, I finally figured out he was calling to find out what time I was making him dinner.

July 1, 2014

I have been in Nashville the past few days, getting some writing done and having a little bit of a break from my folks. Though I worry constantly, and I have been calling them three times a day to make sure they are all right.

I keep thinking that I shouldn't have come down here, but Dad seemed to be pretty good. I'll be home on Saturday around suppertime and am hoping that they can keep themselves fed and alive until then.

Of course, as soon as I landed in Nashville, I was getting messages from friends that a tornado had touched down about an hour outside of Calgary. I phoned home to check in, and Mom told me the weather had been so horrible the big dogs ripped the moulding off the door leading from the garage into the house, because they thought the end of the world was upon them. She let them come and lie down on the kitchen floor and took my little Midi upstairs to their walk-in closet.

"Why did you go upstairs, Mom. I thought when a tornado is coming you're supposed to go into the basement?"

"I just thought Midi would like it in there."

"I thought you were finally out of the closet, Mom."

That made her laugh. "Well, I guess not. . . ."

Mom has also been giving me daily updates on Midi's bowel movements, which she delivers in a flat, newscaster's voice that makes me laugh every time. "She had a big poo, so that was good." Or, "Dad took her around the yard to poo, but he doesn't know if she did or not, I guess we'll find out."

Mom always says, "There is no news around here," and then proceeds to tell me a long list of things that seem to be of great importance to her.

She and Dad have had the TV stuck on Fox News since I left. "The remote quit working," she told me, which means that my dad probably pressed the wrong button and then kept pressing buttons. I don't even know how to start telling them how to fix it. It's one of those universal remotes that are supposed to be able to tell you what to do if something goes wrong, which is why I got it in the first place.

I don't know what I would do without my friend Donna, who checks on them all the time. Last night she made them chicken and my mom told me it was better than "the stuff I made."

As I hung up the phone from this call, I could hear my dad in the background saying that the goddamn TV was still stuck. My mom began to answer him as she put the phone back in its cradle, and we were cut off. I could picture them in their recliners, staring at that remote control like it was some kind of evil puzzle set by the devil himself.

It's hard being away from home. Not just home I guess, but my family and my friends and my stuff and sometimes my dog(s) and my cat.

I have been travelling for over thirty years for my job and it never gets easier. I have to make sure that I keep up some routines even when I am not waking up in my own house. I have to be mindful of how I am feeling and what I am thinking because it's too easy, when you're away from home, to fall into a slump—not quite depression, but it could turn into that if I am not mindful of how I am and who I am. I don't want to sound like I sleep in a pyramid wearing healing crystals around my ankles, I only want to stress how important it is to keep a watch on how fast you're running around.

I make sure to take time in the morning to simply lie there for an extra few minutes to prepare myself for my day. I don't turn on the TV or pick up my phone. I just take a minute to say to myself that I am going to be okay and that my day is going to be a good one. It may seem like a small thing, but intention is huge. Intentions are what I am made up of. I intend to do good things and that is something that keeps me balanced and serene.

I always make sure to eat something when I first get up, whether that's an apple stolen from the hotel lobby, a power bar, a package of cookies from the airplane the day before, a muffin or a bag of peanuts that's been in my purse for a week. You cannot function without food in the morning.

Another thing I do is sit peacefully for a few minutes to try to sort out everything that's going through my brain. I stop to ask myself how I feel. It may seem silly, but how often do you ask yourself that question? *How am I?* A simple thing, but it keeps me sane.

Travelling is not for the frail or weary.

July 6, 2014

My cat, Sweetpea, is completely blind. I think her hearing is starting to go too. She is nineteen years old, still has pretty great-looking fur, still cleans herself, still spirited even with all her obvious little glitches.

She is, however, peeing and pooping all over the house. I've been putting off the inevitable for two months, torn between having her stay and graciously "letting her go." She loves sitting in the sun. She still loves to roll in catnip—I put out so much for her she always looks like she's covered in oregano—and have her chin scratched. Even though I want her to have one last great summer, the "waste" issue is wearing me down. Though maybe it's partly my fault: I have been giving her a lot of treats and feeding her as much cat food as she wants, whenever she wants.

I know some people would say, "Hey, don't feel guilty, it's just what has to be done." But I do feel guilty. Thinking about having the vet come here to deliver that ever-so-final little prick that allows her to drift off to forever land keeps me awake at night. I feel like I am facing two really bad choices.

I am watching Sweetpea now. She's circling the kitchen floor and bumping into the chairs like a furry pinball machine. It makes me smile, although it's not that funny, especially not for her. She is trying to find her way back to her couch, which I've covered with old bedsheets because she sheds so much. She is having a harder and harder time figuring out where her bed is. I feel like I am watching her decline inch by inch, unable to make that phone call to my trusted vet, my dear friend Judith.

I wish I could find the simple strength to do the right thing. This really sucks.

July 13, 2014

Of course I always knew that my parents would get older, that things would change. But I wasn't prepared for how much they would change and how quickly. It's been uplifting and heartbreaking and mind-boggling watching what a fifty-six-year marriage means to two people when things start to fall apart, and how adaptable those two people have to be.

My parents do this kind of dance in the house, weaving in and around each other without really having to think about who will move where or how or when. It is a dance created over time, through practice and repetition. By this point they read each other through a glance, even a shift in breathing.

"I can tell he's asleep by how he's breathing," my mom will say. "I can tell if he's sick by the way his face changes colour. You wouldn't notice, but I do. . . ."

Last night, my dad was staring at my mom's teacup, which was sitting to one side of her dinner plate. I thought to myself, *What the hell is he thinking about?* My mom glanced up at me and said, "He wants a glass of water." He nodded and looked at me as if to say, "What took you so long to figure that out, you silly goose?"

Through all the anger and disappointment that they've faced, they have somehow managed to maintain a precarious balance of peace between them. Even facing the brutal reality of my older brother being in jail for all these years, they stand in a lonesome solidarity that no one else can even begin to understand. They've never turned any of their lives' calamities into resentment or hatred. These days, couples seem to split up at the first sign of any trouble. My mother has said to me on more than one occasion that she doesn't always like my dad, but she always loves him. That has always made so much sense to me. There are days when I don't like him either, but my love for him is constant.

He is grouchy a lot of the time, and ungrateful, and when he doesn't want to answer a question, completely unresponsive. I end up getting mad, but I look at my mother and she is always calm. "I just ignore him," she'll say to me. "Don't let him get to you." And then she grabs a handful of peanuts and heads out to feed the squirrels who wait for her like she is Jesus returning. They get so excited I always worry about them leaping right into her apron. I watch them rub their little hands together like they're praying, and exulting, "We are saved!"

My parents are the last of a dying breed. There is a joke in there somewhere, and I will figure it out eventually. They are an old-school couple who have made their way courageously through life, never feeling sorry for themselves, finding grace in the small things. And always going forward. No matter what.

One of those small reliable things that hasn't changed with my parents is the simple joy of having a good meal together. It's something they look forward to—my dad especially. I started cooking regularly for them after several trips over to their place to help them to "figure out this goddamn can opener." My dad has always had a way with words. I was marching home in a bit of a huff after opening the third can of chunky soup in as many days—wondering why the heck they were eating so many meals from a can—when it dawned on me: heating up a can of soup was something my mom could still manage to do.

I started by cooking dinner for them once or twice a week. Within a month, they were coming arm in arm across the driveway towards my house almost every evening, chattering away like two old birds chirping on a wire. It was all they could do to wait until five-thirty. If Dad had had his way, he would have been on my doorstep by three.

I hadn't really done a lot of cooking in my life. I mean I cooked, but pretty much the same five or six things over and over again. My job has always meant that I eat out—a lot! Now I had to figure out how to prepare nutritious but fun meals that Mom and Dad would enjoy. Thank heaven for the inspiration of cooking shows. Luckily for me, my folks would try anything I put in front of them and they always seemed to like it. The other wrinkle was that I rarely had the time to spend three hours putting together a difficult recipe, so I eventually adapted many of my favourite dishes so that making them was simple and easy. They really loved my turkey chili (see page 175).

July 18, 2014

When tragedies happen now, they feel both global and incredibly personal. It's like a shard of grief pierces the hearts of people all around the world at the same time and unites us for a moment, crossing all borders, all ethnic lines, all colours and religious beliefs. We are bound together for that moment by an incredible wave of compassion and loss and empathy for people we do not know, but feel a connection with. More than a connection—we ARE those people. Even if it's just for a breath or two, we are those who are lost and we wince with a surreal kind of shock. Who could do this? What makes people so evil?

I walked the dog down the road this morning after a terrible night's sleep. Syria, refugees drowning in the Mediterranean. I listened to the crunch of gravel beneath my feet and squinted into the sun, filled with a dull kind of agony. I actually told Midi, right out loud, that she was lucky she didn't know what was going on in the world.

I couldn't get the pictures out of my head: clouds of thick black smoke billowing up into the bluest of skies, vast fields of grass that had been waiting to be cut, now burning. Such a juxtaposition of everything good and everything bad. Little shoes sitting beside a scattered deck of playing cards, a leather purse, a passport, a suitcase perfectly intact, waiting for its owner to claim it.

As the dog and I walked home with the wind at our backs and the sun streaking through the trees, I thought to myself how good people are. How kind and helpful and hard-working and empathetic. Even though my faith in the human race is challenged at every turn, I still believe that goodness is abundant and that bad people will not be able to turn us into the bitter, hateful souls they seem to want us to be. They want us to be like them, full of dark and dread and doom, to become wicked beings set on causing pain for the sake of pain. I will find the good people and I will surround myself with them. I'll keep trying to be decent and thoughtful and helpful and creative. I'll leave good things behind me when I pass. I promise this to myself.

July 27, 2014

I went over to my parents' house yesterday because they needed me to open a can of ham. My dad thought he had really lost his marbles but, honestly, I couldn't get that f&*%ing can to open myself. I told him it had nothing to do with him, that this time it *was* the bloody can opener's fault. He was *so* relieved. "Well, let's throw it out," he said.

"We can't throw out a perfectly good can opener!" I said.

"Yes, we can. Your mother and I threw out the coffee pot last week, so we can throw this out too."

"You threw out the coffee pot?"

"It wasn't working."

"You should have called me to come over."

"Your mother doesn't want you to think we're crazy."

"Well, it's too late for that, Dad. . . ."

My mom started laughing her head off.

The simplest things are getting complicated. Just when you think you're at an age when you've pretty much got life figured out, you forget what you're doing. You forget how to make the string longer on the weed-eater. You forget how to set the clock radio. You forget how to pop the gas thingy open on your car so you can fill it up.

It's these things that bother my parents most of all, not the fact that Dad can't walk to the mailbox anymore, or that he doesn't sleep well, or that he can't drive his truck. It's not being able to open a damn can of ham.

After they threw out their perfectly good coffee pot, they headed straight over to Walmart and bought a Keurig coffee brewer. They can't figure that out.

A friend printed out a very large set of instructions and taped them onto the cabinet door, and they STILL can't figure it out.

My dad was a person who could have assembled a helicopter if he put his mind to it. He could do or make anything—build houses and rebuild truck engines and make delicate rocking chairs and tables and birdhouses. So it's hard to watch him struggling with a can opener or making a cup of coffee. It's harder still knowing my parents feel ashamed about not being able to figure out those simple things.

"I don't know how you do all that stuff on your phone," my mom said to me one morning. I don't know how myself, to tell you the truth. I just figured out how to change my ringtone a month ago. It had been some kind of minstrel-sounding harp for the previous fifteen months.

Even though they are fighting their way through their own maze most days, they still find humour in everything. Mom was feeding the dogs saltine crackers this morning, right out of the package.

"Are the crackers stale, Mom?" I wondered.

"I doubt it."

"I mean, can't you guys still eat them?"

"I don't know." And then she laughed and got up and walked outside and fed a handful of old cupcake bits and some bacon to the squirrel who had been waiting for her all morning.

August 6, 2014

I finally found the courage to have Sweetpea put down. I went back and forth so many times trying to come to terms with what I had to do. I guess I hoped that one morning I would wake up and find my old cat curled up in her favourite bed, already gone to heaven. But when the weight started coming off her and her hearing went the way of her sight, I knew it was already past the point where I needed to show her some grace.

My mom helped me bury her on a ridge behind the house, both of us crying as we shovelled dirt over that little cardboard box. I'd wrapped her in a fuzzy towel. Then we said a prayer and stood looking out over the river. There were birds singing particularly loud and sweet, just for Sweetpea, I like to think. The wind was warm and slow, and the trees waved back and forth with a slow and steady solidarity, like pallbearers. I hardly slept last night, riddled with guilt, not because I'd finally asked the vet to come but because I have been away so much over the years. Sweetpea was left alone in the house a lot after her two companions died. It was just Sweetpea, roaming around, keeping the mouse population in line. We always left music on for her, a lovely classical mix. Dad would say, "What if she likes country?" I would look at him and shrug and say, "Dad, no one likes country that much. . . ."

Afterwards, when I called Mom to tell her that Sweetpea was gone, she simply said, "Well, isn't it nice to know that she can see again?"

Yes, it is, I said. It really is.

August 19, 2014

My parents left the hose on all night in the front yard so the trees got a *really* good drink. When I mentioned it to Mom this morning, I thought she was going to cry. I told her it was fine, that the lawn needed a good watering. She said she'd just forgotten it was on. It can happen to anyone—a few weeks ago I was watering a new tree near my driveway and forgot the hose was on for six hours.

I try to not make them feel like the world is ending, but it's hard some days. I feel like my voice is raised and my hands are flying around and my body language is saying, "What the hell are you guys doing over here?" I know that worrying and nagging doesn't do anything but make you sick and tired and lacking in joy. I don't want to be that person. My parents are managing pretty well, all things considered. We'll just muddle through this, one day at a time, or maybe it should be a couple of hours at a time. All I can do is somehow find it in myself to accept all the little changes that are happening. I find it comforting on so many levels just to spend quality time with Mom and Dad. Even *I* am surprised by how wonderful it is to simply sit down and share a meal at the same table. I mean, over the past decade we only really had meals together at Christmas and Easter. This is all new for me; for an hour or two, time seems to stop and I feel like it's 1985.

August 21, 2014

I'm about to go on tour, and I keep running through the upcoming show in my head. I picture myself out there on stage as every possible thing goes wrong. My clothes fall off, I forget lyrics, I trip into the orchestra pit, my hair catches on fire, the band goes on stage completely plastered. I worry this way every single time I head out on the road.

The worst hours are between 3 and 5 a.m. After my mind wanders through every possible performing disaster, it moves merrily on to the fragile yet humorous state my folks find themselves in these days. Then I enter the weird zone where I count heartbeats, think about my future, my past—why I never had children, how I am going to die—then count more heartbeats and obsess about a developer who is planning a massive housing project on my beloved road. I run through the entire spectrum of horrors that my brain can conjure up.

At this point in the game last night, I managed to talk myself into getting up and working out, which I SO did NOT want to do. Once I got going, though, I felt better. There is something about sweating out one's troubles that makes it worth it to climb ten thousand imaginary stairs.

After I had showered and fed the dog, I walked over to Mom and Dad's.

Mom said, as I came in, "You look tired. You're kind of a funny colour."

That is always nice to hear.

She knew by the look on my face that she should follow with something a bit more upbeat. "Well, Dad and I thought we could take you to the buffet tonight at the Casino."

I wanted to go back to the funny-colour comment. "What do you mean, funny?"

"Have you been suntanning?"

"No," I said, "I have not been suntanning." Under my breath, I muttered that I could probably manage a buffet even though I was a weird colour.

But Mom overheard me and had a helpful suggestion. "You could wear a hat and some glasses so that nobody would notice."

Thank you. Thank you very much. Wearing a hat and

sunglasses to an Asian buffet at seven o'clock at night never attracts attention.

September 13, 2014

I have been meaning to write for two weeks, but life on the road tends to capture your entire being and hold it hostage. I find it hard to sleep on the bus, even with Midi snoring away at the foot of my bunk. I am envious of her ability to travel so effortlessly. Maybe if I was her size and could fit in a purse.

Even when I was younger, I could not for the life of me fall asleep on a tour bus. Imagine being in a long dark box that is really noisy and pitches from side to side as it barrels along at ninety kilometres an hour.

People always think it's so glamorous on the damn bus, but the bus is like camping without ever being able to stop.

On the day I left, my mom had to call 911 and have Dad taken to the hospital (where else, pray tell, do you take a person in an ambulance?). It was a giant shit show just as I was about to get on the plane, and I was completely torn. But my little brother, Patrick, and his wonderful girlfriend, Jodi, and my dear friend Theresa completely stepped up and looked after everything for me. I am so blessed to have people in my life who are dependable and loyal and trustworthy. I don't think I could have carried on with the tour if it weren't for them. You really do find out who your friends are when tragedy strikes and the ball drops and the bull wanders into the china shop!

Anyway Dad came home again a few days later, thank heavens.

Life really is moment to moment. I know I can't live too far in the future, because it just makes me anxious. I tell myself to deal with where I am and what's happening in the moment. I called

Mom a little while ago and she said Dad was quiet today.
Perhaps he is thinking about life trickling by. . . .

I am literally going to go and get on the stage right now.
That's living in the moment.

October 2, 2014

I made it home last night and it is so very quiet around here. I
had gotten used to being around twenty-four people at all times,
eating with them, sleeping with them (you know what I mean
—on the bus), laughing with them, crying with them, creating
with them.

My band was, as always, brilliant. Keith, Pat, Allison,
Graham, Darcy, Kristyn, Mike—what a dream team. My crew
was amazing too, leaving no detail to chance. I am blown away
by what they do, and how well they do it. Every night I stood
on that stage was pure magic. If you've ever doubted that the
universe has a God, music is a reminder that there is one. I don't
know what that means, or what it is, or who it is, but I am amazed
and humbled by whatever or whoever has put this all together.

I got up this morning and went out to the garden to dig up
my potatoes, onions and carrots. I had to leave them in the
ground when I left for Victoria to start the tour, but they all
survived. I am making Mom and Dad roasted root veggies and
turkey meatloaf for dinner tonight. They both look great and
are in good spirits. When I walked into their house last night,
they both stood up to greet me (which made me want to cry),
then Dad said, "We're still alive!" Then Mom said, "Well, just
barely. . . ." And then we all laughed. Alive indeed.

October 8, 2014

There are days when I feel like I am the worst person in the
world. I sit in a chair and feel like everything I do and

everything I say is mean-spirited and selfish. When it comes to the care of my mom and dad, this is the weight that slithers my way on occasion. Both of them are now all over the place when it comes to their memories and I find myself getting more and more impatient—more snippy, more grumpy, more frustrated.

Mom said to me the other day, "You always seem mad at me, Jann. . . ." I died a little inside after she let that sentence fall out of her mouth. I told her I wasn't mad, that I was just caught off guard with this new version of them.

"This is new to me too," she said. "And I can't do a darn thing about it. I am practically drinking that coconut oil you bought us."

That really made me laugh. I told her that I hoped she was kidding.

But I loathe watching them misplace every single thing: keys and purses and credit cards and hats and coats and money and electric bills and coffee mugs and glasses and the TV remote. There are elves in the house, "movers," my mom calls them, who take things and put them just out of reach, just out of plain sight.

"The movers move things," she said a little while ago. "Either that or your dad and I are going crazy. At least we're doing it together."

They are indeed doing it together. They *never* get mad at each other. My dad will answer the same question from my mom a hundred times and not even flinch. I lash out like a whip after about the fourth time Mom asks me something and then feel completely ashamed. I called her the other day and told her how sorry I was and she said, "About what?" It gave me a lump in my throat the size of a toaster.

"About me being so short with you."

"Well, you're doing the best you can. You always do and we appreciate everything you do. . . ."

When she lets me off the hook that way, I can feel my heart pump the blood to the end of my fingers. I can feel it fill my cheeks and pulse in my running shoes that are tied too tight again.

My mom is so kind. It baffles me how my dad's drinking and carrying on back in the day didn't make her coarse and bitter and unmerciful. No matter how much he yelled, or how drunk he got, or how often he stormed around like a four-year-old, my mom just kept right on being herself: empathetic, good-natured, generous, funny and thoughtful. And here I am, turning into some kind of memory referee, blowing my whistle and crying foul every time either of them repeat themselves or get mixed up.

After much reflection, I have realized how scared I am. I am scared of them forgetting themselves and taking me with them into oblivion. I am scared of how their lives seem to be stolen day by day, their shared past thrown into a blender. I am just scared.

The funny part of all of it is that they aren't the least bit concerned. They don't seem scared at all. They are happy. They are light-hearted and positive and faithful and easygoing. I am the only one freaking out.

I need to tear a page out of their book and just calm the hell down. So what if they put the remote in the fridge? So what if the car keys are in with the dog food?

As Mom said, "We find things eventually, Jann. It's not the end of the world."

October 11, 2014

I spent the afternoon yesterday in the yard with my parents. There was something about the autumn leaves falling from the

After much
reflection,
I have realized
how scared I am.

poplars through the sun, like thin gold coins, that eased my heart. Everything seemed so familiar and easy. It made me think of my childhood, when life was a hell of a lot more straightforward.

My mother did warn my brothers and me about what was coming. She told us one similar fall afternoon, many years ago, that we'd have to fend for ourselves someday, buy our own toothpaste and toilet paper, that she and Dad wouldn't always be there to do everything. We were standing out in the yard leaning on our shovels and rakes. Mom and Dad had us all working in the garden and we hated every second of it.

Yeah, right, I thought to myself. *Like that will ever happen.*

None of us thought it would ever be any different that it was that crisp day. We would be looked after forever. That memory feels like a shard of beautiful glass piercing me.

Yesterday the air was cool enough for us to need our old sweaters and ball caps. Mom was wearing one from 1994 that says "Insensitive."

"You STILL have that crazy old hat," I said to her.

"What hat?"

"The one that's on your head."

"What's the matter with it?"

"It says 'Insensitive.'"

"And. . . ?"

"It's just funny that you still have it."

"I have everything I ever had," she said, matter-of-factly.

And she may be right, because my parents' house is starting to look cluttered. Not terribly, yet, but you can see the wave beginning to gather speed.

The clutter started in the closet upstairs and now it's creeping down the hall into the laundry room. Piles of magazines and all kinds of rags. Hundreds of bits of paper with random things written on them.

I recently picked up a pile that was sitting on the dryer and shuffled my way through it. One note read, "owe jann 19 dollars." It was dated last July. I stood there wondering what she owed me nineteen dollars for.

Mom started laughing when I asked her why she was saving all this crap. She said, "I just need it and I don't know why. So there. You can burn it all when I die."

"Maybe I will burn it, or maybe I'll sell it all on eBay."

"You should just have a big yard sale. You could wait a few months at least after I'm dead. . . ."

"I'll wait at least three months."

"Good."

"Fine."

Then we both laughed and Dad told us we needed to get back to work. And then he laughed too.

We spent the rest of the day gathering up the potatoes and the carrots and onions, rubbing off most of the dirt and putting them down in the root cellar. Dad built it himself years ago and it's still rock solid. I marvel at what that guy could do. Literally anything.

It felt good to get it all done before the winter sets in.

It felt good to see Mom and Dad out in the yard.

I tried to stop time with my head and make the moment freeze. The two of them chatting back and forth, taking exactly one second at a time.

November 1, 2014

As soon as I walked through the door at my parents' place, I spotted Mom's new wallet open on the side table with nothing in it . . . well, nothing but her Indigo/Chapters reward card. For the last three weeks I have been shuttling Mom all over town trying to get all her ID replaced after she lost her purse and had no idea where or why or how ("I think your dad left it at the coffee place. . . ."). I was hoping to find it stuffed in a birdhouse or in the dryer or in the garage or in the dog food bag, where a lot of lost items turn up, but no such luck. Credit cards, health care card, driver's licence, pacemaker cards, birth certificate —everything was gone.

It is no simple task getting everything back, let me tell you. Thank God my dad had their passports tucked away in his sock drawer, because that became my key to being able to replace everything without having to resort to crying my head off at the registrar's office.

So, long story longer, before I left on a business trip last week, I had it all dealt with. I felt a huge sense of accomplishment and relief. I told Mom how important it was to put everything back in her wallet after she used it AND to put her wallet back in her purse. Then I saw it sitting there with nothing in it and I could hear my own voice rise into the air like cheap fireworks. "Where the hell are all your cards, Mom?!"

"What cards?"

"All your credit cards! All the stuff we replaced before I left!" My tone was more an angry colour than a sound.

"Why would I take my cards out of there? I don't remember doing that. I don't know where they are, Jann. They are somewhere, though. I bet they are in my purse."

She started rummaging through all the coats and scarves hung on hooks by the back door. I stood over her like a prison guard and said, "Don't you have someplace you put your purse every day?" Being bossy is unbecoming of anyone, and is not my nature at all. I hate the new me.

As she kept searching through the coats, she said, "It was nice not having anybody yell at me this last month. Your dad's half crazy, but he doesn't ever yell."

I was immediately filled with regret and shame. "I was only gone a week."

"Well, it felt like a lot longer."

She finally found her little red purse and started pulling things out if it. Kleenexes and hand lotion, a comb, more tissues, a toothbrush, a mirror, her cell phone (for which they'd been looking for days), a handful of loose change and finally a little stack of cards. "There, see?" she said.

I felt stupid and small. Again. "Why didn't you put them back in your wallet? You're going to give me a heart attack!"

"You're going to give *yourself* a heart attack, Jann."

"I just don't want you to lose all your stuff again."

"Well, I might. That's just how it goes when you're old. And if I do, we can go get them all again. I can go and do it with your dad—we don't mind. But I found them, so there."

I told her I was sorry, and that I didn't mean to raise my voice. Then my dad came in and sat at the kitchen table and asked me what was for lunch, like he hadn't seen or heard anything that had been going on. I picked up Midi, and walked over and handed her to him. He warmed her little feet in his hands.

"Do you want me to make you some lunch?" I asked him.

"Sure," he said, grinning from ear to ear. "Whaddaya got?"

"Whadda*you* got?"

"I'll eat whatever you want to make me."

"How about alligator?"

"Fine."

"Alligator it is."

Then my mom came into the kitchen clutching all her stuff in her hands and looking all over the place for something.

"What are you doing?" I said.

"Looking for my wallet."

33

I didn't make alligator, but warmed up some of my "stewp" and toasted slices of the cheese and onion herb bread I like to make. (See pages 171 & 172)

November 8, 2014

I was away again this week, and my parents did well. I left Midi with them and I think they would rather have her sitting in their kitchen than me.

I called them every day to check up on the pill taking and dog walking and the meals they were having and how everybody was sleeping and if I had any mail and what the neighbourhood news was. (Dad gets up at two in the morning every night and goes downstairs to sleep in his chair, which is why I always ask about the sleeping thing.) Every day, Mom would tell me that nothing was new around there and that nobody had died. "We're all alive so that's good!" she'd say, and then laugh this adorable laugh, and a wave of relief would wash over me.

Not dead indeed. My parents don't live in the future ever. I seem to constantly be living in a day that isn't here yet. They always deal with the hour they are living in. They don't get ahead of themselves, they don't worry, they don't lament or dread what may or may not be coming their way. I need to get to that place, and sooner rather than later.

And my mom is so funny, she really is. When I call, she always tells me two things right off the top: whether Midi had a poop, and what they had for dinner. The other night she told me that she and Dad split a ham sandwich and that dad's half was bigger than hers. "He can sure eat. . . ." she said and I could hear her roll her eyes. "He ate the last cinnamon bun this morning, too, and didn't even ask me if I wanted a bite!" And then I heard Dad yell at her from across the living room because he always listens to every word she says to me. "I gave you HALF of that bun, Mother!"

"You did? Well, your dad just told me that he gave me half of his cinnamon bun. I guess I forgot." And they both laughed like little kids.

"Yes, you had half of that bun and you had a big piece of my fudge too!"

They often talk back and forth when I call and I just hang on the other end of the line and listen to them chatter.

I said, "Hello, Mom. Do you want to hang up?"

"No."

"Okay, well, you were talking to dad and I just thought you wanted to get going."

"It's the only time he listens to me. . . ."

"Why is that?"

She paused to think that over, then said, "What were we talking about?"

That's when I started laughing and she started laughing. It's always the same.

Sometimes they will both be on the phone in different rooms and things really get interesting. More often than not they'll be talking to each other and I just go along for the ride. I treasure these crazy calls. I feel like I am in some kind of cosmic farce, watching them enjoy each other—one of the secrets to a marriage that has lasted almost six decades.

Good lord. That is something I will *never* experience, which makes me kind of sad. Unless I get married tonight and try to stay alive until I am 112 years old. Um . . . not gonna happen.

November 15, 2014

Yesterday, my dad turned seventy-nine. I told him I couldn't believe he was almost eighty! He said that he still felt like he was a kid. "When I look in the mirror I just see me like I always was. I look the same as I ever did."

He doesn't have one single grey hair on his head and not too many wrinkles either. My mom says it's because of all the rum he drank—it "preserved" him.

I thought about what he said for much of the night. It's only when you see old pictures of yourself that you realize how different you look. I think I feel stranger about the person I used to be than the version of myself that I am today. I always think how sad it was that I actually thought I looked fat in old pictures when I was *so thin*!

Time trickles by and you see your face every single day and seldom do you notice the small and constant changes. I don't anyway. Although I did just spot a wrinkle by my nose that I'd never noticed before. . . .

There is so much grace in even being able to grow old. Sure, getting old is difficult, but *not* getting old is more difficult still.

Last night I had my parents over to my house, along with my little brother and his family, to celebrate Dad's big day. Dad seemed very unmoved by the whole thing. He said, "What's so different about today? We eat over here every day, so I guess every day is my birthday?"

Good point. Every day *is* your birthday. I have never been much of a birthday person, because much like my father, I feel like every single day I am here is a reason to celebrate.

I made pizza (see page 179), because that's what Dad wanted, and a giant salad just to bring a sense of "we are eating healthy" to the get-together. Patrick and Jodi brought some very evil yet delicious cupcakes that were mostly buttercream icing. My mom LOVED them. We also had mini "turtle" cheesecakes that were a big hit. Dad, who has diabetes on top of everything else, had one of each, because "To heck with it, it's my birthday and I am going to be dead someday anyway."

My mom thought it was Pat's birthday most of the day, so we all had a good laugh about that.

After dinner we all sang a bad version of "Happy Birthday" and Dad sang along too, which was classic. These times are good ones. I keep trying to lock the memories away somewhere safe, so the "me" of the future will remember and smile.

November 28, 2014

There's been a bit of a reprieve around here as far as my parents go. Everyone is sleeping well and eating well and enjoying the days. The TV remote has worked flawlessly for nearly a month. Nothing has been misplaced or picked up and carried off by the "movers." Everyone has their glasses, the credit cards are in Mom's wallet right where they should be, the dryer door hasn't mysteriously locked itself for no reason whatsoever. No one has fallen in the yard or wandered down the road or forgotten anything of any great importance.

It's funny how everything seems to ebb and flow, like a tide coming in and going out. Mom and Dad have these lovely conversations that float back and forth between them. It's like little birds fly out of their mouths with messages. They have been puttering around the house, putting a few Christmas things up in the yard, hanging the odd picture, cleaning out closets, pausing for cups of tea and toast slathered with thick sweet honey. It's like we've all slipped back in time about ten years.

I stand at their front door and see life as it was a decade ago and want to burst into tears. It's like Mom and Dad have been given a gift, a pause if you will, in what has been an otherwise exhausting series of crazy events. (For me, not them!)

I saw Mom this morning out in the yard wrapped in layers of coats and hats and scarves feeding the birds. A few days ago she fed them a tray of old cinnamon buns and some cheddar cheese. She is still tying strips of cloth in the branches for the squirrels and all the strips are gone in the morning. Thanks to my mom there are a lot of posh squirrel houses out there in the trees this winter.

I am making us a vat of pea soup for supper tonight (see page 173) and we have the latest installment of the Stallone franchise to watch. No clue what it's called, just that it's got every aging action star from the last four decades in it and my dad will love it.

And my mom will probably nod off. We usually have to pause once or twice for a bathroom break (usually for me, not them).

Whatever this break is, whatever this delicate in-between stage may be, it has me shaking my head in wonder. Perhaps we get a little reminder every now and again of how good things were and can be, just so we can hang in there a little bit longer and don't end up completely mad at God. Or maybe not. Anyway, it's like a pre-Christmas miracle.

The cliché is that we are supposed to live our lives in "gratitude." But gratitude is not something you acquire like a Happy Meal from McDonald's. It's something you have to slowly create in your daily life through intention and sincere acts of goodness and kindness.

You can *say* you're grateful, but are you really? I don't ever use the word lightly. I have realized over the course of my life that gratitude has become the foundation of everything I do and everything I think. It's become a very tangible, tactile force in my music as well.

I do not get out of my bed without taking a moment to whisper, "Thank you." I can't go without saying it or my day loses some of its value.

Bear with me. Gratitude is a way to belong to the universe, a way to attach yourself to everything that ever existed. When grace and thanks and mercy fill your days, you can survive all hardship. You can conquer any wrongs, and you can help others to do the same. Gratitude is my cape, my superhero "must-have" to get me through life. Gratitude helps me to understand my parents and my shortcomings and my failures and my triumphs.

It has changed who I am and how I react to things. Without this magical energy in my life, I feel lost. There have been times when I didn't understand how much I took things for granted, and my whole being felt the effects of that negativity. I do not want to walk into the sunset anymore, I want to run into the sunrise. I am filled to the brim with gratitude.

December 4, 2014

How do *you* feel?

It's hard being a person. The constant barrage of horrific and disturbing and sad and tragic news stories that pop up in front of our faces on our screens is nothing short of overwhelming. We are challenged on every possible level, our emotions tossed from side to side as though we were on a broken little ship lost at sea.

There are days where I find myself sitting in a chair, just trying to articulate *how* I feel. What do I feel right this second? What makes me happy? How am I going to get through the day while keeping my fragile sanity intact? Sometimes I just do not know how I feel.

My mom tells me that it's hard to negotiate the world these days even if you're sane. But how do you do it if you're somewhere on the cusp of sanity? We are all slightly broken. Some of us even rattle when we walk, and God forbid we should ever break into a canter—we'd sound like we were running open-armed through a china shop, knocking over every cup and every saucer and every lovely crystal dancing figurine.

Life blasts at us in billions of images every few minutes and we are expected to sort them all out and put them in their appropriate place in our hearts and heads. I wonder how most of us stay upright, to tell you the truth.

The pettiness of social media astounds me. I have been witness to the crushing wrath of the mob on many occasions over these past few years, seen people tossed away like they were a bit of old newspaper. It's sad that we sit here behind these keyboards and judge others with absolutely no regard to what happens to them afterwards. Victims of sexual violence come to mind. So many women are subjected to shallow and cruel jabs from other human beings who have never even met them, who have no facts to hand, save for the "facts" they have read on the internet, and yet feel compelled to spew their garbage at anybody who will listen.

How women breastfeed their babies, how they dress their dogs, how they dress for a party, what they wear to work, how much they weigh, what their legs look like in a bathing suit, how much cellulite they have, how they raise their children, how they vote, speak, look, act, smell—you name it, and we are there with a quick thumbs-up or a thumbs-down, making damn sure they know how very wrong they are. The insults pass back and forth like a pot of cold mashed potatoes at a really bad dinner party.

There are those that argue that the effect of social media is positive and useful and helpful and you can meet new friends and learn new things and you can "like" a dog or cat rescue, or join forces to ban Abercrombie & Fitch because they don't sell a size 12, or boycott the Russians. There is no end to it, and it's all . . .

Exhausting.

Words are big. They define who you are. They are permanent. I don't think most people realize that. What you say is who you are. So try to be gentle on social media. Lift others up when you can, even if you don't agree with what they have to say. Don't always turn your words into weapons when you can just as easily make them doves.

December 7, 2014

My dad wants to come over here earlier and earlier to have dinner. He called me at ten in the morning and asked me when would be a good time to come.

"Well, at suppertime, Dad."

"How many hours away is that?"

I could hear Mom in the background telling him that he had just had breakfast, for God's sake.

"Today it'll be about seven." I know I sounded, well, kind of curt.

"That's a long goddamn time to wait. Okay, then." I could hear how disappointed he was, and felt bad one more time about seeming so mean.

A while ago he rang my doorbell at 6:15 a.m. I was still sound asleep and at the shrill DING DONG I shot out of bed like a rocket. As I stumbled to the door I was cursing the moron who actually thought it was okay to ring somebody's doorbell at that hour. I threw open the front door thinking I would see one of the landscaping guys who had been putting in sod that week, but it was Dad standing there looking like he'd been up for hours.

"What's for lunch?" he asked and as he was clearly about to come right in, I got out of his way. I was grumpy, of course, but I managed to find the grace to follow him into the kitchen where I ended up making him a grilled cheese sandwich. He didn't talk to me, just sat at one of my stools and watched me make the sandwich. "Want a glass of milk?" I asked, and he nodded yes.

There is something about feeding people you care about that is extremely comforting for both of you. My dad looked six years old sitting there at my counter, his uncombed hair falling over his forehead. He has a hard time keeping still. It's like he has things to do but he doesn't know what those things are. Time to him is just a big mess and there is nothing for us to do but give in.

Despite the complaining I seem to do, I love seeing Mom and Dad coming toward my house at night to have dinner. Mom will call me to make sure it's the right time, usually more than once. They sit at the same spot at the table and wait for me to set their food down in front of them. They both look relieved to NOT have to worry about what to make themselves.

I hadn't planned on feeling the joy that I feel. I hadn't counted on the sense of well-being and accomplishment. The comfort I get from cooking simple food for my parents has come as a lovely surprise.

December 20, 2014

This year my mom didn't bring her Christmas tree up from the basement.

For the past decade, when the season was over, she has simply been draping the fully decorated tree with a giant bedsheet and having it carefully carried downstairs and stored in the corner. It suddenly seemed crazy to her to take all the decorations off every year, only to put them on again twelve short months later. "All Dad has to do," she said, "is plug the damn thing in."

When I asked her why she wasn't bringing it up this year, she just said that she didn't feel like it.

I guess Christmas the way it used to be—the way I remember it—is finally over. I have been having the dinner at my place for the past five or six years, but Mom had always taken the time to at least decorate her house.

She has a little village with street lamps and a church and a preacher and a snowman that all lights up. When I was young I loved looking at it for hours. She'd put it up on the mantel over the fireplace, just out of reach of our reckless fingers. It's sitting in its cardboard box now and I doubt it will ever see the light of day again.

I remember Mom and Dad throwing Christmas dinner at their place a few months after my dad had had a fairly major stroke. (He's had several small ones since.) He had got up at three in the morning and put the turkey in the oven, having stuffed it with a loaf of bread still in its plastic bag. He had sprinkled some kind of spice on it, which we never did identify, and cranked the whole thing up to 475 degrees. My mom smelled something in the night and jumped out of bed to find the turkey burning.

Dad had looked at her with such defeat and shame. On some level, he understood that he'd screwed up and done something that didn't produce the results he had hoped for—which was making us all a Christmas dinner, just like he had for the past forty years.

Later that day, we made a game out of guessing what Dad had liberally spread all over that poor turkey and had a good laugh. Dad said, "Pepper . . . lots and lots of pepper, I think . . ." and then he laughed too.

This whole entire thing is about love and understanding and failing and getting up and trying over and over and over again to be the best version of ourselves we can be.

I guess Christmas the way it used to be—the way I remember it— is finally over.

December 24, 2014

Another year went slipping past us like a raindrop down a window. I remember on this exact day last year I was sitting right where I am now, reflecting on the previous 365 days of life's adventures.

Life ain't for the faint of heart. You have to wake up each and every day and realize that you can and will begin again. It doesn't matter if you've screwed up or lost your way or made giant mistakes or failed or fallen, you can always keep going forward.

You're not supposed to get it right out of the gate. My favourite people in the world, my dearest friends, all rattle when you give them a shake. They have little pieces that have broken off inside of them that are a constant reminder to them, and me, of how far they've come and how much they've learned and what they have survived.

The human spirit is unstoppable. You are an intricate part of everything that has ever existed or ever will exist and *that* is fucking fantastic. No matter what else is going on.

December 26, 2014

Small changes gather speed and weight, then join together and get big without you really noticing it happening. And then you're faced with something like making the *entire* Christmas dinner at your house.

I mean, I'd been asked to bring a salad or a casserole, but never the whole turkey dinner—stuffing, gravy and all. But when Mom and Dad couldn't manage a big family dinner anymore—it was too confusing and far too complicated for two people who were both well into their respective battles with memory loss—I had to step up.

I remember the last Christmas dinner my parents attempted to put together. Dad was still able to drive back then, and they had picked up groceries, which they both loved to do. They bought all the things that one would need for a holiday feast. And there were still plenty of carrots and potatoes and onions from the garden—thank God, because that year we needed them.

Everything seemed to be in pretty good shape except that my parents had bought a five-pound turkey for fourteen people. I didn't even know turkeys could be that small. It was Christmas Day and there wasn't anywhere we could buy another bird. Dad looked as though he was going to sob and I did my best to tell him that everything was going to be fine.

I called my brother and told him to bring a ham and I peeled another pot of potatoes. I figured everybody could have a small piece of turkey, a slice of ham, and two pounds of potatoes and carrots.

We didn't have any stuffing, but we did manage to have a whole lot of laughs. I think that was the same year Mom made her famous cheesecake and we had to eat it out of bowls because it NEVER set. We laughed our heads off eating liquid cheesecake.

January 7, 2015

I had a breakthrough of sorts a few days ago, right after I had a mini break*down*.

I'd asked my mom if she thought she would ever forget me and she said, "Well, my brain might, but my heart won't." Those eight words took my breath away. I felt a weight lift off my shoulders that I'd been carrying for the past few years.

It got me thinking about technology, oddly enough. I sat in my old red leather chair, right by the window overlooking my cluttered deck. It was strewn with shells from the peanuts the squirrels and the blue jays have made quick work of since November (I need to clean them up . . . I am becoming my mother, ever so slowly). The sun was streaming through the snow-covered spruce trees as if the beams were gliding in along a ruler, and I marvelled at their perfect geometry. But I digress. I was thinking about the "Cloud"—the Cloud that we are forever upgrading and meticulously monitoring to make sure all our files and pictures and contacts and *stuff* are kept safe and sound so we can find them again and look at them and remember.

Every thought we think, every memory we keep, every fond moment we experience and so eloquently recall as we forge our way through life, is important. They define who we are and why we are and where we've been. Our thoughts, our experiences, are what make us. Having said that, as I watch my parents lose those precious pieces of themselves, I wonder where those lost memories go. Surely they go somewhere?

I want to believe there is a celestial Cloud, hanging like a fly strip in God's porch, collecting every single thing we have ever done or said or thought or seen or heard or tasted. It's all there, stuck to that strip for eternity. We never lose it. It's saved forever. *We* are "saved."

My mom and my dad, and your mom and dad, and every other beloved person, dog and cat and bird and creature—they are all safe and sound and intact. What is forgotten here on earth will be saved.

Always.

January 28, 2015

I have had many days in my life where my room felt like an ocean and my bed nothing more than a tiny ship being tossed around in complete nothingness.

I have experienced hundreds of hours in various states of worry and anxiety and hopelessness and doubt and fear.

All of this anxiety and depression is part of being a person. There is nothing more valuable to a human soul than time spent going through one's own mind and evaluating this thing called life. You're not supposed to be happy every waking moment of every single day. You're not a one-dimensional static entity—you are a constantly moving, evolving, growing, expanding body of energy. There will always be growing pains. Our souls are forever outgrowing our physical bodies, and it hurts our hearts and heads. It's bound to. Or we're stuck, and that hurts in a different way.

Depression can be managed. It can be put in a safe place, enabling a person to go forward with grace and even joy. It has to be managed, though, and that's the tricky part. You have to keep the lines of communication open with friends and family and professional helpers. Isolating yourself can be counterproductive.

Yes, it's great to be alone in order to dive deep into who you are and what makes you tick, but we are social beings. We need each other. We need that connection and that feeling of belonging, even if it's a few hours a week.

"Hope is the thing with feathers . . ." said Emily Dickinson. Feathers are the best flyers in the whole wide world.

I got myself up and out of my funk by making my comfort soup, which is pulled chicken noodle (see page 174). Enough for my folks to take home and have for lunch the next day.

March 22, 2015

I am not even sure where to start. In a very short eight weeks, *everything* has changed. I haven't slept in days. This has been the hardest thing I have ever been through, no contest, and that includes a couple of severe heartbreaks and monumental personal failures of every kind.

Okay, so here's what happened. My dad had a heart attack five days after I left for a five-week tour. From the hospital, sadly, he went directly into a long-term care facility in Calgary. My mom's memory has failed so badly and his medical issues are so numerous that we simply could not keep him at home. The long list of what we've been dealing with: dementia, diabetes, kidney failure, heart failure, mobility, incontinence and high blood pressure.

Before I left, I'd hired a full-time companion to help my parents with the basics. Even though they had their own unique coping skills, their own unique dance, they were sliding into unsafe territory. With me gone, I knew they'd need extra help with meals and driving (Mom lost her licence three weeks before the tour was to start), laundry, simple organization and so on. Then Dad was taken to the hospital and my mom began a rapid mental decline. Removing him from her life's equation brought her house of cards tumbling down.

He was her everything. Even though she was the caregiver, he was her lifeline. She hasn't danced alone in fifty-eight years and it must be completely traumatizing to have had all of these sudden changes in every aspect of her life. It has been remarkable and frightening and fascinating to observe. I feel like I am standing on a sandbar in a strong current where nothing is certain, nothing is static, nothing is normal. I haven't cried at all, which is surprising. I feel like I am so busy trying to put the cards back into place that I haven't had the time.

My mom, always so strong and steady, sits sobbing into her tiny hands. She is filled with what looks to me like pure terror. She resents the fact that I had to have someone come to stay with her. No, she *hates* it. I am completely torn. She can't be alone anymore and I can't be there all the time. I thought she would like the help and the company, but she doesn't. Not at all. I pray that changes.

I hope we find our new normal soon. I hope that the sea we have been thrown into calms a little so we can reinvent ourselves. This is hard, but this really is life. And even a battered, hopeless spirit can find a way to keep going.

I think Mom will rally. I think Dad will be okay away from home. I am relieved that he has twenty-four-hour care, and that he is safe. We plan on bringing him home a few nights a week once he gets settled. I am taking him a bunch of little things this afternoon—throw blankets and an extra pillow, tissues and toothpaste and soap and salt-and-pepper Kettle potato chips as per his request. Some things never change.

I told Mom this morning that I was so sorry that she was sad and that I wished I could do more. She looked up at me and said, "Sad? What was I sad about?"

You just have to stay in such a moment and let it seep into every pore. Onward.

March 27, 2015

I am taking my mom to Germany with me tomorrow. I have a job there next week, which I am so grateful for, and the company I am working with was gracious enough to let me bring Mom along with me. I cannot fathom being separated from your partner of fifty-eight years and learning how to be a new version of yourself. My mom told me it is like "little deaths" every day. Made my throat pinch ever so tightly. But she is forging on.

She was feeding the birds yesterday in her nightgown, apron, and giant down-filled winter coat that had belonged to her dad.

"That's quite the outfit you're wearing, Mom," I said.

She laughed. "I don't give a crap what I look like. . . ."

And that made me laugh. Why should she care? I am twenty-six years younger than she is and I don't care anymore either. At some point, you have to claim your life and cast all doubt aside. It's simply too hard pleasing anybody else.

Today I thanked my mom for having me. She asked me why I was thanking her and I said, "Because you were giving birth to me fifty-three years ago and you said that I almost killed you."

"Well, you did almost kill me, but that's okay. We survived."

We did survive, and then some. She told me my head was so pointed from being "stuck" in there that she kept a hat on me for a year.

That's my mom. She pushed me out into the world and dared me to succeed. She gave me her bravery, for sure.

April 7, 2015

It's never easy watching someone you love slip inch by inch down the rabbit hole. The more I think about it, the more sense it makes to me that Mom and Dad would come unravelled at the same time. They did everything together, and this trip into the unknown is no different. Even though they are physically apart, they will go towards whatever it is, hands clasped. It's their journey and all I can do is try to comfort them along the way. I can't save them from it, that's for sure.

The German river cruise with my mother was a gift, although she thought we were on a train trip. Since we could see the shore blur past us, I guess she assumed we were rolling along on tracks. I corrected her once and then caught myself when she was talking about it again: why do I need to tell her where she is and what she is on? I have to stop being the memory police, stop needing to be right all the time. It's exhausting and completely selfish.

I am going to make her one of those personal photo book thingies she can flip through to remind her of our first-ever trip alone together (unless you count the time we drove to Cranbrook for my brother's murder trial twenty-three years ago—but I digress). This trip was a hell of a lot more pleasant than that one.

The first night on the ship, I lay there in my little single bed and watched her across the room breathing in the dim light. She looked nine years old. I felt tears rolling down my temples and sliding slowly into my ears, making everything sound round and numb.

She said my dad's name out loud in the dark, several times, asking him to come to bed. "Derrel, Derrel, come to bed." It was haunting and life-affirming all at the same time. It took me hours to fall asleep. I was waiting for her to whisper secrets. . . .

Every morning I would lay out her outfits and help her get ready. I had never done that in my life and it kind of scared me. She'd gaze at the clothes draped on the bed and say, "Is that what I am wearing, Jann?"

"Yes, why?"

"I was just wondering. Does that go together?" She pointed at the socks that were black with gold stripes. "That doesn't go together."

"Does it matter, Mom?"

"I like matching socks. . . ."

I changed them to white.

As she pulled them over her bony little feet she said, "It's hard being a mother, isn't it?"

I nodded and had to turn my back so she couldn't see my face curl up into a ball.

My mom was graceful with everyone, quick with a smile and an outstretched hand. I was so proud of her. She outwalked half the dames on those inland excursions to wine villages and castles, climbing steep and crooked stairs with ease, not even out of breath while women half her age had to stop midway up and huff and puff. She never once complained about the rain, either—well, maybe once. She was in awe of everything. In the moment at all times, because that's where she lives now. That's where I need to live.

Dad is managing in the care centre. He talks endlessly about coming home, and it just about kills me. We'll start bringing him home for suppers and sunny afternoons in the yard, but not just yet. They have advised us to wait a few more weeks, until he's better settled. I can understand that. Anyway, we are inching forward.

Mom told me yesterday that summer seemed so short this year. I told her it hadn't come yet and that made her smile madly. "It hasn't?"

"No, it's supposed to be spring, but it snowed again."

"Well, see, there are some good things about losing your marbles. Here I thought we were in store for months of this lousy weather!"

She turned around with her bucket of peanuts and continued hiding them one by one up in the trees. She likes to give the squirrels a challenge.

April 12, 2015

The care facility called me yesterday to tell me that Dad had tried to escape. "Not to worry," they said. "We caught him before he got to the road. We're going to keep a better eye on him."

Apparently he went out a back door and down the alley on a beeline for home. He can hardly walk, so I can only imagine what "beelining" looked like for him.

It doesn't surprise me. No matter how long he will be living at his new place, he will be trying to get back to us. It's heartbreaking and heartwarming all at the same time.

Mom said she fully expects to look out the window one day and see Dad coming through the gate. "He could make it out here, Jann, he's that determined."

All of us have some sort of homing device at the very centre of us. We want to go home, always home, back to where we belong. Life is about belonging for me. Belonging to something, belonging to someone, belonging somewhere. No matter where I go, no matter how far I am across the globe, I am pulled back by a giant elastic band that is wrapped around my body a million times. Home. I know that's how Dad feels. His elastic is constantly pulling at him.

It's weird not finding Dad in his chair when I walk over to their house. He sat in it so much his head practically wore a hole through it. The chair just sits there now like something lost. There is something creepy about a chair that belonged to *one* person being empty. I want to set it out in the trees where we can't see it, but I know my mother would have a fit. Even though she says she doesn't like looking at it, she still wants it there in the middle of the living room.

I keep reminding her that Dad won't be coming home to sleep anymore. I don't want to lie. I don't want to make up some story that will make her keep wishing for him. It's not right. I don't lie to my dad either. When he asks when he will be coming home, I tell him that he will come to spend the afternoon and have dinner, but never to sleep. I tell him that those days are over. I simply cannot lie. It's not fair on any level. People may disagree with me, but I can't do it.

Mom is doing a little better every day, so that's a relief. She has the big dogs sleeping in the kitchen every night now so they are in heaven. They make her feel safe. I figure they will slowly make their way upstairs to her bedroom. They are good dogs, though, and I don't know what we'd do without them.

Mom told me that she was pretty sure they'd just let the burglars through the front door and show them where all the treats are. That made me laugh. Without laughter, all is lost.

April 24, 2015

I was talking to a friend of mine this morning about feeling like I had become orphaned because my parents couldn't continue on in their roles the way I wanted them to. I keep trying to drag the past forward, like some giant sack full of stones. I want them—I *need* them—to be who they were. I can hardly pull that sack behind me, but it doesn't stop me from trying.

You have to let it go. I know that. I have to let my parents become who they are going to become. I have to make it easier for them to go forward towards their own destinies. I cannot change what is going to happen to them.

Change is a hell of a thing. I have to find some sense of grace for myself and not be repeating old behaviours over and over again. This has been the toughest time in my life, for many reasons, but I am getting a lot better at crying my head off. I am getting a lot better about getting really mad and howling at the moon.

May 18, 2015

I feel like I have been living someone else's life these past two months. I stare at the ceiling in the middle of the night (which I can't really see because it's pitch black in my bedroom) and wonder how everything changed so quickly. Just a few months ago my life was completely different and the change makes me profoundly sad. It hasn't just been my parents, but also a million other things that have shifted around in my life and left me with a feeling of helplessness.

Still, Mom and I and my cousin Tracy (who drove all the way from Lethbridge) went into town to see Dad yesterday at the care centre and he seemed better than he had in a long time. When we got there, Dad was just waking up from an afternoon nap and he looked like he had a squirrel on his head.

Mom, of course, had to comment on that. "Derrel, what did you do to your hair?" She also asked him where his tooth was. I told her that his tooth had been gone for ten years and she was gobsmacked.

We have had this same conversation several times. A few weeks ago it went like this:

"Where the heck is your tooth, Derrel?"

"It's been gone a long time, Mom," I said.

"Well, that couldn't be possible! Jann, I stared at that head for fifty-eight years and he had a tooth in that spot."

"Well, I am telling you that his tooth has been gone for at least a decade. Don't you remember him spitting water through that hole to impress us with how far it would go with a little effort?" I couldn't quite believe she didn't remember that classic move. It was really something to behold.

"No, I don't remember one single thing about him spitting water through a hole in his teeth."

Dad sat on his bed and watched us talking like he was at a tennis match. He hasn't asked me to take him home with us for over a month. It used to make me feel like crying. I felt so guilty. I still feel guilty. I think the decision to move him out of the house will always haunt me a little bit. I know it was the right thing to do but it doesn't make the ache in my heart any easier to deal with.

But after the initial shock and grief, my mother is doing better without him at home. Not having to look after him twenty-four hours a day has reduced her stress. Her memory hasn't gotten worse. She doesn't repeat herself as much and she is sleeping better and laughing more. She is eating better and seems a lot more herself.

She was going down with the ship, as it were, and now her daily life is so much more manageable. Even she says she is glad she isn't having to deal with him all day long, though she feels guilty too.

We still see Dad almost every day and his overall health has improved as well. Getting his meds on time and on a consistent basis has been big, as is having constant companionship and help with mobility.

We are slowly getting to know the interesting people who live there with him. Betty, who has rollers in her hair every second of the day, and who is forever looking for her room. The "where is my aunt and uncle" lady who repeats that question for hours on end. The other day Mom said to Dad and me as we passed by this lady's wheelchair, "Would it kill you two to be this poor woman's aunt and uncle?" Dad laughed out loud.

June 3, 2015

We brought Dad home for the first time on Monday. I talked to him the previous afternoon and told him to be ready to go in the morning. I also told him that I was going to make him mow the lawn when he got here and he laughed a little bit. He has lost a fair bit of weight, perhaps twenty pounds or more. It worries me, considering that according to the staff at the lodge, he doesn't ever miss a meal. Mom says he is "dwindling away." She is the only one I know who uses that word, other than my gram. *Dwindling*. Good one.

When he walked through my front door he started to cry, which made my throat shut immediately. He seemed overwhelmed by everything. He kept saying that it all seemed changed and different.

He can hardly walk now. Between the dementia and the blockages in his legs, he can maybe stumble a few yards at a time. We all grabbed an arm and an elbow and guided him over to the kitchen table. He wanted a Coke and his cup of coffee, which he had brought with him. He tried to talk but didn't really manage to get much out. He just blinked ever so slowly and looked carefully at our faces. I wondered what he was thinking about.

He was very calm and reflective. Like he was somehow living in slow motion while the rest of us were stuck on fast forward. I wanted to slow down too. I wanted to crawl into his head and watch the movie he was watching. My mom sat beside him and kept looking at him like he was an apparition.

"Are you tired?" she asked him and he nodded yes. We put him on the couch and Mom untied his shoes and set them beside him on the floor. That too, made my throat squeeze nearly shut. It's the smallest things that set me off. It's the tiniest details that make my heart swell up like it's been stung by a thousand bees. You realize that things don't matter. Not the chairs we're sitting on or the mugs we're drinking out of or the clothes hanging off our shoulders. None of it matters. My dad doesn't care about his things anymore and to tell you the truth, he never really did. The man owns two pairs of shoes. He used to laugh at Mom and me and tell us that we could only wear ONE pair at a time. My mom would tell him that that wasn't the point!

I could tell that he wanted to go "home" after he had his hot dog. I don't know how to feel about that. The idea of home changes for all of us I suppose. It's a place in the heart not on the map.

June 21, 2015

Father's Day has always been a bit of a quandary for me. I find myself on this particular Father's Day both guilty and, sadly, indifferent. Lots of people will be spattering the internet with glowing "I love you, Dad" banners and reminiscing about the times their fathers took them to baseball games and on fishing trips and whipped up barbecues on sunlit decks, and all those wonderful things that dads do.

That was never my experience with my own dad. He was an alcoholic for most of my formative years. My strongest childhood memory of Dad is of him screaming at us. He was the worst kind of drunk, the kind who had to be right, and liked to intimidate everybody around him. If we didn't bow to his every whim, we suffered the consequences.

Thank God, he was hardly ever home, because when he was around he was angry, he was brooding and he was always looking for a fight. My older brother got the worst of it. My dad picked on him constantly and I don't know why even to this day. Dad has never talked about it. Since he stopped drinking he's held his past as far away from himself as possible. Some of us would call that denial. . . .

I didn't realize that we weren't really a "normal" family until I was about thirteen. Mom would warn us not to bring other kids home from school "just in case your dad shows up."

How she hung in there still defies reason. "I did it for you kids," she'll say now and then. "I don't regret it."

It's funny how the difficult things in life can force you to go in certain directions. Had I not been wanting to avoid his frequent wrath, I doubt I would have sequestered myself in the basement, where he never came, so I could learn how to play guitar. Music became my refuge, my safety zone, the place where nothing bad ever happened, the situation I could control.

Don't get me wrong—my dad taught me countless, invaluable lessons. He didn't take any crap from anybody and, believe me, that rubs off on a kid. I remember how people reacted to my dad when he was determined to get his way, whether it was demanding another cup of coffee in a diner or his money back on a pair of pants that didn't fit. To this day, I don't tolerate nonsense in my business life. I expect people to be fair and ethical and decent. Period. If they're anything but that, they won't be working with me.

Seeing my dad now, in his room in the care centre, a mere shadow of his former self, is very hard. The man I used to be afraid of is now a meek and mild, helpless child. I was thinking about how much resentment I have been carrying around and how much I don't want to still be carrying it. I want to let it all go. Maybe today I'll start. I dragged it with me because I thought I needed it to protect myself. Silly what our hearts and minds do to us.

Even though he had his own struggles and his own demons, my father provided for us always. Even though he battled depression and addiction and failure, he managed to teach us important things, like working hard, and not giving up, and being your own person. He always showed up to help the neighbours build fences or move furniture or dig postholes or round up a lost cow or pour concrete driveways. He never stopped working and he never stopped being hard on himself.

I didn't always like my dad, but deep down I have always loved him. It's hard being a person. When I glance back at him as I walk out the door after a visit, that love resonates like never before. So I guess it's not indifference.

July 4, 2015

It's hard how much things shift in the course of a few days. One of the most difficult things for me to get my head around is how much my mom can change even over a few hours. She can seem very clear and very much herself and then in the blink of an eye, she is gone: the person I've known for so many years leaves the building. I find myself feeling very resentful and bitter about this. I don't know how else to describe it. I get angry. I feel like somebody broke into my heart and took my most precious thing. My mother.

I don't know if I am mad at her for leaving me to fend for myself, or if I am mad at myself for being an asshole. I have a hard time being patient and being understanding. I fight the urge every single day *not* to be the memory police and constantly correct her. I so badly want to be mindful of living where she lives now and not expecting her to be where I am. That is no longer possible, certainly not on a full-time basis.

I know that, and yet I fight it constantly. My mother has been such an incredibly positive presence in my life. She has shown me, rather than told me, how to be a decent, empathetic human being. She's not overly sentimental or protective, but she's been a loving force behind me, whether I've succeeded or failed. I was an idiot over a period of many years . . . I truly was. Some people say they have no regrets, but that isn't me. I have many. Yet my mother has always told me that I punished myself far more than she ever did, or would, and that is certainly true. She was the first person to ever tell me that I needed to learn to be kind to myself. When I was a kid, she rarely scolded me—she'd just have to look at me and I'd realize how far away from being my true self I was acting. I hated letting her down.

She worked full time when my brothers and I were quite young, so making meals and doing chores were mandatory for us kids. I appreciate that so much now. As much as I *hated* helping around the house, I am so glad that she had the backbone to demand things from us. She expected us to show up for our own lives and to do good things. She was my mother and my mentor, *not* my friend. Friendship would come later, when I was old enough to appreciate what a friend truly is.

My mom still soldiers on through whatever life puts in her path. I have never heard her complain about anything, and I am not exaggerating. She doesn't complain. I have never heard her speak ill of another human being, either, except for my dad when he really deserved her wrath. I am in awe of her fortitude and steadfastness. She's fair and good and she can laugh at the worst of times. She has laughed us all through so much grief and loss.

But memory loss kicks everything and everyone around it in the balls, pretty much. The mother I knew is slowly going away. When she reappears, it's for shorter amounts of time. I feel alone and I want to blame somebody.

Right now she is losing track of what time it is, and getting up earlier and earlier. Sometimes she'll call me at six in the morning and ask me what I am doing and then she'll ask me what *she* is supposed to be doing.

"What do you want to do?" I ask, startled awake and with my heart pounding because I think something is terribly wrong.

"I don't have a clue," she answers cheerfully.

"Have you had coffee?"

"I think so. I can't seem to get over the time change."

"What time change, Mom?"

"I'm not sure . . . just the time change. I can't get used to it and I can't find my glasses."

"Did you check in your bed? You've been making your bed lately with your glasses still in it."

"Did I make my bed?"

And so we go, around and around, until I end up walking over to her house and finding her glasses and checking to see if the coffee is on and the bread is out on the counter.

"Did you have something to eat?"

"Yes, I did! I had some of that cake Deanne made me!"

She's so excited that she remembered she had cake, although Deanne is actually Nadine and I am actually the one who made her the cake. It's all I can do not to set her straight. It's all I can do to not sit at the kitchen table and bawl my head off.

August 18, 2015

I haven't written anything in a long time. Life has a way of picking you up and dropping you off a few weeks later at an unknown destination. Some days it really does feel like I've been plunked down in a strange land surrounded by strange people and strange things I hardly recognize. My own house feels "funny" when I've been away for a while. Autumn is already nipping at the flowers and the grass is slowing down. Right now even a change of seasons is unsettling.

My dad is fading away. Literally—he's lost forty pounds in the past six months. The weight is falling off him like it wants to go somewhere else, anywhere but where his body has found itself. He looks at me like I have an answer to his quandary, when in fact, I do not. His unhappiness is palpable.

They moved him to a more aggressive dementia wing of the facility because he had become combative with the staff, verbally and physically. Now he's basically strapped to a wheelchair for the entire day. Before they started tying him in place, he'd struggle to get up then crash to the ground like gravity was his lover. It was bad. It was constant. He was injuring himself and they were concerned for his safety. I understand that. They told me they had no choice but to strap him down, but he is miserable.

I've been on the road for work these past few weeks and when I saw him today, it was shocking. His face has changed so much. It made my eyeballs hurt trying to keep the tears from shooting out like bullets. I know he's dying, an inch at a time. I can't tell you how helpless we all feel, watching him slither his way down into the earth. I pray at night that he will go to sleep and simply not wake up, but the world doesn't work that way.

I guess he still has work to do here on planet Earth. It doesn't make it any easier to think that God has a plan for my dad. It doesn't make the hurt and pain and angst and worry one little ounce less. Watching him go is hard, but that's what people do. They make their way out of this world the best way they can. One breath at a time.

August 31, 2015

I am sitting in the Chicago airport. I'm trying to get home. Dad is barely hanging on. He was unresponsive when they rushed him to hospital. Pneumonia. Another little stroke. Low blood pressure and racing heart. The man is worn out.

My little brother, Patrick, has been with him night and day, along with Jodi. Dad's two sisters and his sister-in-law came up from Lethbridge to see him yesterday. Mom has been there, too. Pat and Jodi brought Mom to their house to sleep while I've been away.

Every damn time I go away that father of mine gets himself hauled off to a hospital. Perhaps he likes having me frantically trying to get home to him. Still, looking after Mom and Dad for these past five or six years is the best thing I've ever done. The lessons learned have been too many to count, and the value beyond priceless. Caring for people makes you better. Period.

I hope I get home in time to say goodbye, but if I don't I have a great sense of peace. I stopped being mad at him a long time ago. I started forgiving and I started letting go of all the things that didn't really matter in the long run anyway. Funny what finally makes you let all the hurt and anger go.

August 31, 2015
With Dad now.

August 31, 2015
Dad passed away at 8:15 p.m. We love you.

September 1, 2015
Oh, what a day. I feel like I am tangled up with all these loose ends that life has decided to gather up and hand to me. Here, life says, untangle all these little puzzles and get back to me when you've figured it out.

Every thought in my head has a hundred layers. Layer upon layer of pain and confusion and disbelief. It's like the world decided to test how much chaos it could inject into my heart without it stopping. And my heart keeps going. The blood whirls around inside my chest like a tsunami, gathering up every memory and pushing them all out my tear ducts. I try to keep myself from crying and I don't know why. It actually, physically, hurts my jaw *not* to cry. I don't know why it's my jaw that hurts—that's just where the pain ends up.

People are buzzing around me, saying important things, and I nod and say things back to them like: "I don't think I have ever seen or heard anything so terrifying as my father gasping for air on that tiny bed. . . ." And then I wonder if I said it out loud or if I just said it in my head. I am pretty sure it was in my head because they are asking me how I am doing and I don't even know because I feel like I am on mute. I am adrift inside my breaking heart.

I kept telling him to go. I remember that.

I was thinking that it was taking so long, that he was working *so* hard to get out of himself. His struggle tore me and my little brother into shreds of something we couldn't even recognize.

I kept looking across the bed at Patrick and whispering, "Where is the peace? Where is the fucking peace?"

It never showed up.

Not until that last unusual moment.

A strange noise crept out of his lungs like it was embarrassed. Dad looked straight up and finally left his body there, in the blue-and-white cotton gown that had probably been worn by a hundred other sick and scared people.

I felt like I died too.

We all did.

I thought for a second that I felt him pull at my sleeve, but it was only my heart beating so hard that it was moving my arm up and down ever so slightly.

Part of me wishes I hadn't seen any of it, that I could have just remembered him walking away from my house, arm in arm with Mom, carrying their leftovers.

But I stayed in the thick air of that little "comfort" room for him.

Because I knew he was scared.

September 17, 2015

It's been a couple of weeks since Dad went off on his new adventure through time and space. His wooden urn now sits on my kitchen counter, watching me walk around each morning with my hair hanging down. We haven't decided what to do with him. I think he is happy here, though, although he doesn't say it outright. . . .

I will tell you that it has felt like a storm pouring down emotions. One minute you're up and the next minute the discomfort is agonizing. Anxiety has tiny little teeth and they nip at you with great persistence. I can't describe the blanket of fear that folds itself over me at times. I can hardly breathe, and then it lifts as if it was never there at all. Funny.

I wish I knew when it was coming, though, because I would lock the doors and close the windows. But I don't, and simply have to go through it. You can't skip the hard bits in life. I feel ridiculous even writing this, because what are my hard bits compared to the troubles going on in this world, the profoundly horrific things people face every single hour of the day: the war, the hunger, the violence, the loss, the hardship? My troubles are little invisible things that God doesn't have time for. Nor should he take the time . . . I know that. No matter what happens in my life, I am filled with gratitude.

Two days after Dad passed away, Mom was officially diagnosed with Alzheimer's. Her condition has been a blessing in a sense, as she has seemed to deal really well with everything. The disease somehow tempers sentiment, at least at this stage — that's what I have found, anyway. Of course, she's very sad, but it's manageable. I think had he died four or five years ago, she would have been flat on her back with grief. She tells me she forgets to be sad. She is still somehow very funny, perhaps without knowing it.

For instance, when she and I drove home from the hospital after Dad had gone, it was very quiet and eerie in the car. We were both processing the hours and hours of his labour: death is much like a birth. At one point, Mom turned to me and said very calmly, "Well, I can't believe that you had him put to sleep, Jann." I just about drove off the road.

"Put to sleep? I didn't have him put to sleep, Mom!"

"I saw you give him that needle."

"I would never do that! It's illegal for starters."

A few more minutes went by as I could feel her thinking hard about everything. Then she turned towards me and said, "Did Dad give you permission to have him put to sleep?" Her hands were folded on her lap, her fingers twisted like tight bits of rope.

"Mom, he died of complications from a lot of things. He was so worn out and tired and fed up. . . ."

"I saw what I saw. . . ." she said. She was convinced that I had him put down.

I wanted to laugh but it felt completely inappropriate. When I think of it now, though, it makes me smile. In all that sadness, the absurdity of what she was saying to me somehow erased the pain for a moment or two. I knew at that moment that we'd would stumble along somehow, and figure it out one small thing at a time.

October 8, 2015

My mom amazes me every single day.

October 9, 2015

Anxiety is new to me. You'd think that after fifty-three years on the planet I'd be well past having new things happen to my body, but I guess I'm not. My own flesh seems to be in revolt against me.

One minute I'm sitting here minding my own business and the next minute this thing wraps my torso like a python and decides to squeeze the ever living hell out of my heart and suffocate me at the same time. It's beyond scary.

I kept thinking I was having your mid-life garden-variety heart attack. My instinct was to sprint around the house in

full-on panic mode while attempting to dial 911 and then run out
into the middle of the yard and start yelling for help while I was
waiting for the ambulance to arrive. I didn't. The rational part
of my brain kept reminding me not to believe what I was
thinking and told me to stay put and keep breathing in and out.
So that's what I did. I shut my eyes, concentrated on breathing
in and out, and told myself I was okay . . . over and over again.
I didn't expect it to work, but it did.

For the time being.

Anxiety doesn't stick to a schedule. It's its own boss and it's
the worst boss I've ever had.

After that first assault, I was on full alert waiting for the
python to come back when I least expected it—when I was
walking through the mall or sitting on a plane thirty-eight
thousand feet in the air or walking the dogs or eating soup or
watching a movie. I was ready and waiting for something that
may never happen again and that pissed me off. It pisses me off.

I have learned that anxiety loves it when you sit still and
worry. It hates it when you engage with friends and laugh out
loud and get fresh air and keep moving. It hates it when you
don't give up and when you're creative and insistently filled with
hope. Anxiety doesn't let go of you easily but that doesn't mean
you can't be in the same room with it and still get stuff done.

October 28, 2015

It's been two months since Dad died. I moved him in his little
mahogany box to a spot in my living room. We are going to
figure out where to lay him to rest in the spring. There were so
many decisions to make when it first happened that we simply
haven't gotten around to it yet. I think he likes it here in my
house. Mom always says that she can't believe that they fit all
of him in *there*—she points at the urn. I don't comment.

It's all still weird in a thousand different ways. I'm not really used to the idea of never seeing him again. Mom, however, says she sees him all the time.

"He was in the cupboard above the sink in the bathroom last night, Jann, and he looked SO young!"

"The cupboard?" I said, lifting an eyebrow.

"Yes. You don't believe me but he was there as plain as day. He looked really good."

"Does he say anything to you?"

"Not a word. He just looks at me for a while and then he disappears."

I love having these conversations with my mom. They make me happy from the inside out. I don't know if it's the Alzheimer's, but she sees him and it's as real as anything. I asked her if she was scared when he showed up. "Not one single bit," she said waving her hands through the air. "Why in the world would that scare me? We were married forever."

"Well, it would scare the living shit out of me, Mom!" And it would. I would run out the front door screaming if my dad showed up in my bathroom cabinet to stare at me.

Still, part of me is a little bit jealous that she is able to see him —and that she has such an open heart and mind that she's not the least bit freaked out by seeing a dead person in her bathroom. She says often that she just forgets to be scared. I need to forget to be scared too.

November 22, 2015

I have my mom propped in her favourite chair watching a Western with Gregory Peck. She was agitated when she got here at 7 a.m., but she's settled down a bit. Her disease is stealing her sleep and her sense of reason and her sense of self.

For the first time, I can see the paranoia slipping in and out of her mind like a thief, stealing memories.

We've spent the last few hours going around and around in a giant circle and I'm exhausted. My mom doesn't know she has Alzheimer's. How could she know? She doesn't know why I have the Christmas tree up. She asked me this morning if I needed help taking it down. I told her we hadn't had Christmas yet. She looks at me, perplexed, then tries to cover her tracks. Her mind is busy trying to hide its problem. The mind is so tricky. It constantly re-configures, rewires, reroutes, trying to protect itself from what it knows.

I can't imagine how maddening it must be for her. I mean, I get so anxious I feel like crying most of the time. The disease is taking me over too, even with the help I have. None of that changes the fact that I am losing my mom, an inch, a thought, a memory at a time.

She just told me she doesn't want "those ladies" in the house anymore—meaning the lovely souls who help me at night because Mom can't be alone. She says she doesn't need them because she is getting better. "I will beat this," she says. I just mumble, "Okay. I hope so, Mom." And then a few seconds later, she tells me that she hates being alone in the house.

"That's why the ladies come in the evening, Mom."

"Oh," she says, nodding. And around we go. . . .

I tell her that I love her more than anyone in the world and that I am making decisions for her that I know she would be making for me if I was in this shape.

"I am sick of you telling me I'm sick," she says sternly.

I tell her I am sorry.

Then she says, with a smile on her face, "Should we take the tree down?" She loves to be helpful.

"Why don't we leave it up for a while?"

"Until New Year's?"

"Sure, New Year's would be good."

"I wish you didn't have to go away all the time."

"Me too, but we all have to go to work."

"Maybe I'll retire. . . ."

"I think you should retire. You've been working for fifty years."

"I have?"

I laugh, and we go back to the top of the same pile again. And then I make her my favourite pancakes (see page 166).

December 11, 2015

I feel like I'm making good decisions for us most days, but of course, there are times when I feel like I am completely lost in the fog. Mom now gets very anxious at some point during every day. Mostly in the mornings when she walks over to my place. She struggles with having "the homeless people sleeping on my couch every night." She means the women I've hired to make sure she's never alone. Nadine and I have decided to order a "bed chair" for the office so the "homeless ladies" can nap in there, where she won't see them first thing when she wakes up. Mom told me this morning that she is doing her best to look after them, which made me want to bawl. Her heart is so big.

She also told me that she wanted to be normal again and I told her why in heaven's name would she want to be that? I told her normal was for the birds. That made her laugh. I am getting better at moving her away from an issue that she has fixated on. I talk about really abstract, fun things that distract her from thinking about her troubles. It has to be so difficult trying to make sense of everything that darts around her mind. I can't imagine. Perhaps one day I too will experience this dreaded thing, this loss of self.

Mom misses her independence more than anything. "I just want to walk down the bloody road and get the bloody mail, but I can't seem to do anything without those people trailing behind me," she says. She hasn't wandered off anywhere yet, but I expect that will be one of the things that will come eventually. We head back to the doctor on December 16 and I told Mom she could ask him any questions she might have about what's happening. I told her we could write them all down. "Fine," she said. "I've got a few things to tell that guy!"

We have lots of laughs every day, despite it all. Mom had a cataract operation last week and told me afterward that she didn't think that she and doctor saw "eye to eye." She can still be so witty.

I guess I assumed that at some point Alzheimer's people would know what was happening to them, but they don't. She doesn't, though she did tell me that I needed to get my brain checked too. I agreed.

It broke my heart today when she said, "I feel like I am sitting in this house waiting to die." I should take her somewhere in January, give her something to look forward to, even if she forgets what that something is.

I do feel sad a lot.

It's hard to lose your mom a bit at a time.

It's weird and frustrating.

Sometimes she is *so* there, and I cherish those moments. I hate seeing her cry. She'll tell me she doesn't even know why she's crying. I don't think it's important to always know why.

December 20, 2015

My mom always wants to do something for me, to help in some small way. She never wants to be idle or just sit on the sidelines while life is going on around her. I hate to admit this, but from time to time I feel like I take advantage of the fact that Mom likes to mop and vacuum. I may have her run over my floors more often than they really need doing. . . .

But in my defence, it keeps her busy and more than that, it makes her *happy*. Mom still wants to have a purposeful life, to be wanted and useful. She can fold a basket of tea towels for an hour and not be the least bit bothered, in fact she'll tell me how much she enjoyed it. She loves wiping counters and watering plants. Although it's very difficult for her to stay on task. She'll have a potato peeler in one hand and a potato in the other and still have to ask me what she's doing. Then she'll peel that potato down to a nubbin if I don't keep an eye on her. I usually have her stir a pot of soup if I have it going, or slice up an onion. Onions can be cut into any shape under the sun and they'll work just fine in a recipe.

I think she misses cooking a lot, because she wants to be in the kitchen as much she can. I am always trying to figure out what she can do without setting something on fire or cutting off one of her fingers. I am getting better at just letting go of details. Details don't matter. I'm the only one bothered that the tasks she does can be repetitive; she doesn't care how much she does any one thing.

I'm trying to help my mom feel as normal as possible, even if it's a bit uncomfortable for me. Being around food and helping to prepare it makes her feel like a regular person. She can peel a carrot for an hour for all I care now, whatever it takes to feel purposeful is what it's all about.

Tonight we have company coming, and she cut up all the onions for the finger food.

January 3, 2016

You died in the early evening on the last day of August, Mom's birthday—making extra sure we'd remember you on that date, year after year. Like we would ever forget you. I still struggle with you going the way you did. You were not the least bit peaceful, Dad. Not a single one of your last breaths came and went without a lot of effort on your part.

You didn't want to go. You said as much, dozens of times. You were afraid of dying and I don't want to be afraid like you. When death comes over the horizon to take me back to wherever I came from, I want to find some small thread of bravery hanging off my sleeve.

Your death was loud and raspy and the whole room seemed to be under water. None of us could breathe, either. You and your spirit filled every single corner with heaving booms. I thought my head was going to blow off. The pressure was massive. You were in my bones, Dad. I felt you pushing through my flesh like a bullet.

I'd never watched anybody die before and, sometimes, I wish I didn't have that memory of you in peril burned into the back of my retinas. I sometimes wish I had not been there at all . . . but then I catch myself. Patrick reminded me that we were there for *you*, to keep you company, to carry your fear for you.

But even so, you didn't find it easy to go. There's got to be a lot to do when at last the spirit separates from the body. Last little details that have to be attended to. Pacts made with God and the spiritual cleaning up that comes with having been on the planet for eighty years.

Years of diabetes and kidney failure and heart attacks and infections and strokes, and in the end you died of pneumonia.

Mom kept saying, "He's had it, Jann. He's tired. . . ."

She kept asking Patrick if the nurses could at least give you a cough drop. Pat looked at me and shook his head. "She doesn't know he's dying. . . ." he said.

"No, she doesn't," I said.

And then you went. You made a sound that I will never forget. It was part moan and part holler and part lament and part cry and part cheer.

Yes, a cheer.

Finally split apart from the 160-pound body that was keeping you from the abyss. From the wonder. From the glory of the unknown.

I should have stayed with your body longer, afterward, but I couldn't.

Pat pulled the covers up around your neck and kissed you on the forehead and we walked out into the bright lights of the busy hospital.

February 27, 2016

I was so used to having Mom and Dad around, both emotionally and physically—they lived fifty feet from my door for nearly ten years. I have been able to hire enough help that Mom can stay in her house, which has been wonderful for her and me. But she can't be alone anymore and she hates it. *Hates* it. The Alzheimer's dilemma: stay in your own house, but have people there with you all the time, or go into full-time care and *never* be alone again. It's the only way I can get her to understand that we have to have the ladies around. It could be so much worse, I tell her. But Mom keeps saying she wants to be normal.

"What do you mean normal?" I ask her.

"Like other old people."

"Other old people are in nursing homes, Mom."

"No, they're not."

"Yes, they are."

"Not all of them are."

I tell her she has memory problems and that's why we need the help. I try to never use the word dementia, or Alzheimer's. I don't

She can't be alone
anymore and
she hates it.

want to scare her. On some level she still thinks she is perfectly fine. I asked her what year it was. She told me it was 1912. That was the year her mother was born: a date cemented into her brain.

Who is our prime minister?

"That little twerp—the son of that other dead guy."

That made me laugh. She knows who it is, and I didn't need to hear the actual name.

What month is it?

"It's May," she says matter-of-factly.

"It's actually February."

"Good God, you mean we have *more* winter coming?"

"I'm afraid we do."

"Well, that's terrible."

"Tell me about it."

"Tell you about what?" she says, smiling. I realize she's kidding around with me.

We go back to the topic of the ladies in her house.

She thinks they are all homeless, and complains that one of them does laundry non-stop. I joked that maybe I should bring my dirty clothes over and she could wash them too while she was at it. Mom thought that was funny, though not super funny.

"I think she is doing an entire family's laundry, Jann."

"Well, at least she's clean."

"That's true," Mom says. "I couldn't have a dirty person in the house."

"You have a muddy dog in the house every day."

"I don't care. Belle's allowed to be whatever she wants."

"Don't you get tired of all the dog hair?"

"I don't notice it. I don't focus on those kinds of things. It's a waste of time."

Indeed.

March 27, 2016

I'm sitting here with Mom, who is eating a giant piece of my birthday cake and drinking the last few slugs of her Budweiser. My pal Chris ordered me a gorgeous cake that was a work of art and I didn't even want to cut into it. But yeah, we *did* cut into it and then devoured the whole first tier. It's probably the closest I'll ever get to a wedding cake.

My little brother and sister-in-law took Mom to church this morning and she told me that it was "too religious" for her liking.

"But church is supposed to be religious and it's Easter after all."

"No, it's not supposed to be religious. It's supposed to be inspiring and uplifting with a positive message. This was just a bunch of nonsense. There were no songs and I didn't like the preacher."

"Did you have lunch in the basement afterwards?"

"No, because they've given a lot of people food poisoning."

"Damn nuns."

"There weren't any nuns." Mom shovelled another forkful of cake into her mouth. "They are just normal women."

"Damn normal women."

Humour is ALL.

Laugh at all the heartache.

Laugh at all the pain.

Laugh at all the silly things you thought you did in vain.

Laugh at all the guilt.

Laugh at all the wrong.

Laugh until you can't be anything but true and strong.

May 8, 2016

I am so grateful as I sit here next to my sleeping mother. She is having a nap after a great visit with Patrick and Jodi and their twin boys, Ethan and Ryan. She had her beer early, and so she should: today is her day.

I'm grateful for all the times she dragged herself out of bed to drive us to our hockey practices and our baseball games and our basketball and volleyball and badminton tournaments.

For the thousands of Crock-Pot meals and countless words of encouragement, and for her limitless support no matter how badly we'd screwed up.

For telling me my arms were just right and my freckles were perfect and that I was sturdy and not the least bit fat.

For looking past my mistakes and seeing my potential.

For letting me fail.

For hoping for me when I couldn't seem to hope myself.

For sticking it out with Dad, even when it seemed so dismal and pointless. For picking us all up even when she was down.

For inspiring all of us with her determination and bravery.

I have a good mother, and her voice is still what keeps me here.

Feet on ground

Heart in hand

Facing forward

Be yourself.

I loved those Crock-Pot dinners, I even worked up one of my own (see page 184).

May 22, 2016

I have no idea what to do some days. Change is a giant boulder crashing down a mountain. You have to get out of its way or get flattened, but I keep trying to stand in front of it because I'm so scared of what's about to happen.

Does our memory define who we are? Is that the only measure of a life lived? Or is it something much more delicate and written in the stars—stored on God's "Cloud," as it were. I think it might be. But we depend on remembering what we've done in order to navigate our days. We depend on remembering every small insignificant thing in order to define who we are and what we are. Still, when we lose the ability to know what we've done ten minutes ago, or ten years ago, like Mom has, we ourselves may be able to adjust somehow, but the people around us are hit hard.

For the most part, Mom seems unbothered by what she's lost. She is angry with me, though, because of the people I have hired to help us. She doesn't think I'm being fair or caring in regards to what she wants, which is to be on her own in her house. It just kills me that she's mad at me. I am wound up constantly.

"You just wait," she said as I walked her home last night. "You have no idea how terrible it is to have homeless people in your house." She looks at me in a way that I have never seen her look at me before. Her mouth is pinched in a straight line and her brows knitted together. Her contempt is palpable. It takes my breath away. The women try to stay out of her way, sticking to Dad's old office at night with the baby monitor, but she gets up all night long now, and they need to get up with her.

"They're not homeless, Mom. They're helping us. I don't know what else to do. You can't be alone here anymore. It's not safe for you. I'm doing what you would do for me." This sounds reasonable in my head. Like it would make sense to her. It doesn't.

"I would *never* do this to you. Why in the world aren't I safe? This is ridiculous and I'm moving away. I'm selling everything and moving to a country where I can drive."

"Wouldn't you miss us?"

"Well, I suppose I would, but I can't live like this. This is so awful." She glared at me and let out a long sigh.

"I'm sorry, Mom, but this is the new normal. We just have to be grateful for everything we have. I want you to be able to stay in your own home."

"Are you threatening me?" she said, and stopped in the driveway to face me.

"No, Mom. I just want you to stay home and in order to do that we have to have help. I can't be here with you twenty-four hours a day." I wanted to cry but I didn't.

"So you're going to ship me off if I don't have these bloody ladies in *my* house?" The way she looked at me, it was just not the mother I knew. I tried to breathe through it and not lose my temper. I told her that it was all going to be fine and that we had lots of good things to look forward to. I changed the subject. I talked about Midi and how much stuff we have to get done in the yard. I talked about going to Palm Springs in the fall and or going to England to see Downton Abbey someday.

"That would be nice," she said and we started walking again.

June 18, 2016

It's been an incredible week here in Maui, writing with Bob Rock. And, yes, that's his real name. He is one of the most naturally gifted musicians I have ever had the chance to work with in my life, right up there with Ed Cherney and Russ Broom. We've managed to write four pieces of music that may or may not end up on a record, but the process is what always boggles my mind. To create something out of nothing brings so much joy—it's indescribable. It's like a lightning bolt that strikes and makes time itself come to a screeching halt.

The hardest part, of course, is having to be away from Mom. I've spoken to her every day on FaceTime but she always ends up holding the phone up to her ear so I never get to see her! And she sends me texts from her iPad (with a bit of help from Nadine, I'm sure) that are always one very long word.

Hijannmidihadapootodayandwewwntotheriverandbroughtrockshomefor thegardenloveyouandhopeucomehomeeventually.lovemomm

They always make me so happy. (Well, actually, I feel like bawling when I read them because they're so damn sweet.)

Now I don't even remember what I was talking about. . . .

Oh yeah—music and how fantastic it is for the soul. Music saves me every day.

July 18, 2016

Mom told me the other night that she was going to sue me when "this is all over." Lord, have mercy. She is getting really paranoid and thinks that everyone and their cat is out to get her. The other night she walked over here with my grandmother's old mink coat and told me that "those women were trying to steal it." She wanted me to hide it in the basement.

That same night she came back with a jar of pennies and nickels and dimes and said that she'd split it with me. "There's a few thousand in there that we could use for a trip. . . ."

I could see the companion care worker, Sheri, standing on Mom's front steps and watching where she went, kind enough to give her space and let her walk over here. I'd been sound asleep when she rang the doorbell and I almost went through the ceiling.

It makes me sad.

All of it. The changes and the challenges and the weird things that get put on repeat in her head. She is constantly on the move. She never stops. She folds laundry and walks and putters and moves objects and sits up and looks through the trees for imaginary people. If I didn't have help, I would sink so far down I'd never come up again.

The hardest part, still, is that she is so often mad at me.

She looks at me with such hatred that it takes my breath away. And then it passes, and I see her bubble to the surface of herself again and I wonder how my life got to this place. If you'd told me two years ago that I'd be here, I wouldn't have believed it.

And yet, we fall into so much laughter, feel so much insane gladness and joy. It's such a contrast from one minute to the next and it teaches me constantly. It makes me stronger and humbler and more empathetic and caring and kind. At least I hope it does.

It's just life being life and you've gotta embrace it all with your heart pounding away on your sleeve and a smile on your face . . . and don't forget to cry, because that'll get you through anything.

My mom says tears are God's lubricant to get you through the tight spots. That's a good one.

August 2, 2016

Grief is a strange thing. It has an actual palpable weight that makes breathing arduous and seems to stifle the heart. At night the weight increases tenfold and pins you to your bed like an unwanted lover.

This whole past year, grief comes and goes like a bratty teenager, oblivious to any kind of caring or responsibility. It moves around in my body silently, like a cancer. I come up for air every few days, to see the sun, to return calls and make meals for my mother, and then I seem to slip back into dull melancholy. It finds cracks in my armour and burns me with the end of its cigarette.

Losing people is what happens to humans. Like a constant

drip of an old tap. To try to avoid that loss only leads you to avoid true happiness. We die. But as Snoopy always said, you only die on one day. On the rest of the days you live.

When you don't argue with grief like a drunk husband, much good can come from its stillness. Reflection is so important, time alone, solitude, reckoning. You can't be your best self when you're submerged in useless busy-ness.

Most people choose not to stop long enough to think about how they feel. Most people move from one relationship to the next, one habit to the next, one job to the next, one friend to the next. But in my opinion instant gratification leads you down a lonely path.

Change is taking hold of me and morphing me into a much better version of myself, and that morphing comes with some discomfort. And yes, sometimes it feels like I'm being crushed by that boulder.

Instead of telling that discomfort to go away, I'm going to invite it in. I've learned that it seems to not really like that. It's more used to people who hide from it.

I say let fear and grief sit at your table. Talk to them, give them a cold drink and a sandwich. They simply want to be acknowledged and not ignored. When you ignore them, they just hang around longer.

Mom told me a few months ago that there was an Indian man with a baby in her closet. She said he came and went for a few weeks.

I wanted to say, "Mom, there is no man with a baby in your closet." Instead I asked her what he wanted. She told me he said he wanted to go home.

"What did you say?"

"I told him it was that way. . . ."

"And then what?"

"Off he went and he hasn't been back since."

Feel things. Don't be afraid to feel things. That is the whole entire point of all of this.

September 5, 2016

Fall is my favourite time of year, mainly because it's when we start seriously harvesting the garden. All that waiting for everything to grow is finally over. We dig up potatoes and carrots and beets, and if we're lucky rescue a few bright purple cabbages that the moles always try to eat before we do. Both my parents loved working in the garden and between them they had a wealth of experience. My maternal and paternal grandparents kept tidy gardens and some of my fondest childhood memories are of wandering along the rows of peas and eating them fresh out of the pods or eating them pods and all. Mom loves working in the garden with me. She loves watching things grow and she loves weeding. Who in their right mind loves weeding? It always amazes me that she can still recognize the difference between the weeds and the vegetables. She can wield that hoe with the precision of a professional gardener. She doesn't shy away from physical labour—in fact, she thrives when she is using a little elbow grease.

Today we dug potatoes for hours, it seemed. I kept having to make Mom stop to take little breaks. I mean, I was exhausted, but she was like the Energizer bunny. I don't think she has any idea how resilient she is. Watching her work in the garden today brought back so many fond memories. She seemed like her old self, the version I still miss, the one who knew all the answers to my questions and solved all the world's mysteries.

We were both pretty pooped by the time we came in, though.

September 12, 2016

After we adopted Lucky the rescue cat I couldn't believe the difference she made in all our lives. I am gobsmacked by how much my mom's focus has shifted from worrying about myriad things to one dear old overweight cat! Lucky sleeps with her every night and they both just *love* it. I'm not really sure who rescued who. . . .

I have read things over the past several years about the importance and value of pets with Alzheimer's patients, but I didn't expect the cat to have such a profound impact on our situation. Lucky seems to know that Mom needs a little extra attention and is more than willing to give it. A noticeable amount of pressure has lifted off my shoulders and I feel better too.

My goal is a simple one: to keep Mom as happy and as safe as humanly possible. She laughs a lot these days and cries much less. She's walking like she's been a Sherpa all her life and eating like a lumberjack, and that is more than I hoped for at this point. I know it will be a lot worse as the weeks and months go by, but for now, Lucky the rescue cat has brought so much love into our home—and a very healthy dose of hope.

September 28, 2016

People talk about "living in gratitude," but I wonder how many of us are able to truly live our day-to-day lives being thankful for what we have. Like the fact that we are alive and on this magnificent planet, that in this vast universe, we are here, breathing in and out on a tiny speck of wonder, soaring through the cosmos.

I marvel simply looking at my hand. I marvel at tears rolling down my face, at the intricate ability to feel pain and triumph. I marvel at the concept of love, its infinite power, its endless good.

Living in gratitude

is about HOW

we see things.

WOW. (Mom pointed out the other day that WOW was MOM upside down.)

Living in gratitude is about HOW we see things. Your intentions hold incredible power. Be mindful of them. Point them in a good direction. Be earnest. Be the kind of person you want to attract into your own life. Humility takes incredible strength.

And although this life is filled with enormous grief and sadness and challenges and depression and loss and death, it is also filled with promise. We easily lose sight of that when things go sideways, and they often do. Life is going to be hard a lot of the time and that's okay. You can do it.

Living in gratitude involves a lot more than saying you're grateful. It is a way of existing. In poker you often hear the phrase "all in." Living in a real state of gratitude means just that: every second has to be *all in*. Being grateful for pain lessens the hurt. Being grateful for loss may not make any sense, but it's a way of allowing your heart and mind to let things go instead of dragging them with you.

It's interesting to me how much I gain from letting things go, how much I learn that is directly linked to how often I fail. Every single time you don't get it right is like a building block to becoming a better version of yourself.

Flying is falling.

We spend so much time worrying about dying, and that causes us to worry about living. So let the universe have its way with you.

You are a piece of it all. Infinite. Boundless. Indivisible.

October 5, 2016

I had a really difficult evening with my mom. Every week it seems we enter a new phase of this incredibly cruel disease.

More and more frequently, she brings up the issue of people

stealing from her. It's almost always about money. Ten days ago, she wandered over to my house at close to midnight, rang the doorbell and, when I answered, handed me a plastic bag filled with rolled-up toonies. (My dad must have had them stashed in their closet.) She told me the homeless ladies were trying to steal them and asked me to hide them, which I did.

A few days later, she told me they were gone, that someone had taken them. I reminded her that she had brought them to me to keep.

"Oh yeah. I seem to recall that."

"We'll take them to the bank so they're safe." I thought that would make her feel better, but nope.

"The banks aren't safe."

"They're safer than my house."

"Why do you have my money?"

"You brought it here for safekeeping.

I won't bore you with the remaining thirty minutes of the conversation.

Last night she told me—again—that she didn't want any ladies in the house anymore. That she used to like them but not since they've been stealing from her.

The *coins* again. (I need to add that her fortune in toonies amounted to about $200.) She is fixated on them. She goes over and over it in her mind, how all the money she has to her name has been stolen from her.

Alzheimer's pounds all sense into nonsense.

I reminded her that she'd brought them to me a few weeks earlier and that we were going to take them to the bank at some point.

"Are you saying that I am crazy, Jann? How stupid do you think I am?"

The blood rushes to my face and my heart picks up speed.

My feelings are hurt. I know they shouldn't be, but I can't separate my idea of Mom from this version.

"I'm not saying that for a second!" My voice rises and I start to swallow a lot.

Mom becomes frantic. "Why in the world do you hate me SO much?"

I am trying to stay calm but I'm getting angry because I'm helpless, and I know she will forget this whole conversation in five minutes. "I don't hate you at all! I would never, ever, hate you, Mom. You just forgot you gave me the coins. I would never steal them from you."

She sets the dinner I've just made her aside and says she's going home. "I don't have to put up with this!"

"Mom, please sit back down and eat your dinner."

"I'm moving to Vancouver."

"Won't you miss me and Midi?"

"Yes. Yes, I will." Her brain clicks into another gear. "Is this chicken?"

"Yes, it's chicken and the potatoes are from our garden."

"Did we plant a garden?"

"You planted it with me. We had a good day."

"We did have a good day. It was a nice day for it, wasn't it?" She cuts a piece of chicken off the bone and gives it to Belle, our big dog. She pretends that I don't see her do it.

"That's for you, not the dog, Mom."

"It won't kill her to have a piece of chicken."

"You're right, it won't."

"I can't have those ladies at my house anymore. They'll have to find another place to live."

"Okay." What else can I say? My heart is still pounding.

I miss my mom, desperately at times, but even so I'm glad to have this version of her still here with me. I'm trying to learn how to find a language between us that doesn't infuriate me and hurt her feelings. It's like a dance. A dance with music that changes its beat every few seconds.

Mom stops talking now as she often does. She's silent a lot of the time—unless her brain puts her on that crazy-ass spinning wheel. I give her a big bowl of Jell-O and she asks me if I made it from scratch and I tell her, no, that it came from a box.

Then she asks me if it's 1915. I tell her it is.

"See," she says. "I'm not that crazy. . . ."

October 28, 2016

I am a mother to my mother. It's a massive learning curve, not only because I didn't have children of my own, but because there isn't a handbook telling me what I should or shouldn't be doing. Alzheimer's is a different disease for every single person it inhabits. Everything is a trial by fire.

My biggest enemy is patience, or rather, the lack thereof. I feel myself crumble as my mom's memory crumbles. I feel part of myself die a little bit more every time she forgets something new. It's as if we are still joined by the cord that connected us all those lifetimes ago.

Last night when she was here for dinner, she got up and said she had to use the washroom. She made her way over to the door to the deck and was trying to go outside. I asked her where she was going and she said, "I'm trying to get to the bathroom."

"The bathroom is this way."

"It is?"

"Don't you remember the little side bathroom?" I got up and walked her back toward the bathroom door and she acted like she had never ever set foot in that part of my house before.

I feel part of myself die a little bit more every time she forgets something new.

"Well, this is a cute room," she said, looking around. She had her arms folded across her chest.

How, from one day to the next, can things simply disappear?

"Have you always had this?" she said to me with an eyebrow raised.

"Yes."

"Have I used this bathroom?"

"Yes."

So I am a mother to my mother, and I don't know what I'm doing half the time. I don't know if I'm doing the right thing or the wrong thing, making things better or making things worse.

I lost my temper a few hours ago. Mom decided to take the leather straps off the dog bag I carry Midi in. I don't why she thought she needed to do that, and she doesn't know why either. But I can't use the bag without the straps and, more aggravating still, I had just had them replaced. I huffed and puffed and stormed out of her house and across the driveway to my house with Midi under my arm in the bag with no straps. I was being impulsive and bratty and stupid, and I knew I was, before "WHY DID YOU TAKE THE STRAPS OFF?!" even came out of my mouth. I saw her head drop and I wanted to stab myself in the eyeball. I'd hurt her feelings and for what?

Donna, another of our care workers, told me that she would look for them. "Don't worry," she said. "We'll find them."

And they found them two minutes after I'd stomped out the door, sitting on the kitchen counter.

I told Mom how sorry I was a dozen times. "Would a thousand dollars make up for it?"

And she kidded right back, without missing a beat, "How about five thousand?"

November 26, 2016

I don't know my mom very well anymore. I hate even writing down these words. I hurl myself back in time to find scraps of who she used to be wandering around in my early memories.

Emily Dickinson wrote a poem well over a hundred years ago and its haunting opening verse reads:

Pain has an element of blank;
It cannot recollect
When it began, or if there were
A day when it was not.

I can't remember the day when my mother starting becoming someone new, someone changed and altered. I can't remember that precious moment when I started saying the longest goodbye of my life. I wrote a song about it a few months ago with Bob Rock and I'm still having a hard time listening to the demo.

When I was away these past two weeks, I felt riddled with guilt and I felt so relieved at the same time. It's nearly impossible to have these two very different emotions mingling inside my heart. They fight with each other like a married couple on their third bottle of wine. Emily goes on to say:

It has no future but itself,
Its infinite realms contain
Its past, enlightened to perceive
New periods of pain.

New periods of pain indeed. I watched Mom as she napped on my couch last night. I needed to feed us something but I was tired out from travelling. There wasn't a lot of choices. I still have yet to grab a few groceries (maybe tomorrow).

I ended up throwing some spaghetti in a pot of boiling water and dumping on some canned tomato sauce for us to have for dinner—not one of my better creations.

The TV was on in the background and Midi was snoring. It was just one of those moments that I locked onto.

I stood there in front of my sleeping mom holding our crappy supper on a tray and I was torn between letting her rest and feeding her. I wished that I could stay in that ONE spot forever. I wished that I could stay in the quiet and the calm, where this *thing* wasn't going to get worse and that my mom didn't have to endure the indignity of forgetting who she was.

When my dad was still alive, I remember Mom calling me for the millionth time to come over and fix the remote control for the television. I rolled my eyes and told her that I would come over as soon as I could. (I live one hundred yards away, so not a big deal.) When I got there, they both looked at me like I was going to beat them up, and that made me feel terrible. They had heard the anger in my voice and they felt bad that I'd had to interrupt my writing to come and help them. (I'm an asshole.) Anyhow, they handed me an old remote for a TV they didn't even HAVE anymore. I found the right one in the bag of dog food.

You gotta laugh.

Mom said to me, "Jann, you're the only one freaking out. We would have found the g.d. thing eventually."

Very true. I was and am the only one freaking out. My mom is mostly calm and funny and loving life. She doesn't know what she has and I'm grateful for that.

Finally, I woke her up and said, "Dinner is served!"

"That looks wonderful," she said smiling.

I'm trying to focus on what I have, and not what I don't have.

December 15, 2016

When we weighed Mom a few months ago, she was only 104 pounds, and her doctor basically said that I needed to get her to eat, and it didn't matter what—she needed to eat everything. I wish I had a doctor telling me that: "Jann, we need you to eat whatever you want, whenever you want. It's for your own good!" I don't think I'll live to hear those words. It's been challenging, to say the least, to put some pounds on my mother while trying to drop some pounds myself.

A lot of people send me articles about things that might be helpful to me and Mom, especially in the dietary department. I've lost track of how often I'm sent some info on the magical benefits of coconut oil, for instance. But what the heck, I started using coconut oil on everything, eating the stuff by the boatload. It tastes great, it is the good kind of fat and it has a very high "burn" threshold, which makes it great for quickly searing things like fish or onions, or making stir-fries. As far as what it does for memory? That's up in the air. People swear on a stack of Bibles that it makes a big difference in their loved ones who are suffering from dementia and Alzheimer's, so I use it just in case what they say is true. I know that doesn't sound very rational or scientific, but it's not doing any harm, and it might do some good. Mom says to me at least once a week that she thinks the coconut oil is working. It kind of makes my heart ache.

Mom has gained five pounds in the last couple of months. And I'm slowly losing weight: I figured doing something positive about taking care of myself might help me tackle my depression, which comes and goes like a bad relationship. I've been working out hard and eating REAL food, which is exactly what I feed Mom. REAL FOOD. I make sure she has lots of good carbs and I take it very easy on the rice and potatoes and the bread. Otherwise we eat the same things. Eating good food is changing both of us. I have to be at my very best to keep up with this woman.

December 24, 2016

Mom and I are sitting here waiting for everybody to arrive. She is surprised that we are having Christmas *again*. We *just* had it.

We have a few hours to ourselves to drink tea and eat goodies, and she is mowing through the shortbread and caramels and chocolate like there is no tomorrow. We have *A Madea Christmas* playing in the background and every now and then Mom asks me if Madea is a man. Makes me laugh every damn time.

She also keeps asking me if there is anything else she can do. Alzheimer's folks are very task-oriented, or my mom is, anyway. She always wants to be busy and doing things. She wants to be purposeful. Don't we all. . . .

Just now she decided she needs to bring in some firewood. She grabs a couple of logs at a time and goes in and out the patio door. It's quite something watching her can-do spirit. She simply does not stop. So far she has folded clothes, mopped the floor and shovelled the driveway. I feel slightly guilty. No, seriously—I do. It's like having my own personal Molly Maid. I didn't even need the floors mopped, but she was so determined to be useful I couldn't say no.

I totally understand it. I am terrible at sitting and doing nothing. I don't like lying on a beach for more than twenty minutes, for instance, and I'm pretty sure I get it from her.

She finally sits down again and I'm going to try and keep her in one spot for the next hour. It's stopped snowing but while it was coming down it was simply beautiful. She's already mentioned needing to go out and shovel again. You gotta laugh. Maybe it's time to start pouring the eggnog and rum!

I'm so grateful for all the lessons this past year. I'm grateful for the mishaps and the mistakes. I'm grateful for the failures and the heartbreaks and the obstacles.

There is so much joy. There is so much hope.

I truly believe there are a lot of things to look forward to in 2017.

Keep your wits about you.

Be spontaneous.

Be easy on yourself.

Rejoice!

Rejoice!

MERRY CHRISTMAS, HAPPY HANUKKAH!

Whatever your beliefs be, I hope goodness is at the heart of them all.

January 1 at 2:18pm

Hello, 2017.

What are you going to do with me?

I find myself at an interesting crossroads in my life. Well, more of a raging, multi-lane intersection. The last two years have been like watching a slow-motion car crash knowing there isn't a bloody thing I can do to stop it.

We all have times that seem to explode with "happenings" —a succession of years that pound and punch and mete out the unexpected and leave one feeling quite helpless indeed. And then comes the calm, the reflection, the time for the decision making that one has to do in order to turn the chaos into some sort of manageable order.

It's all daunting, but doable.

For the first time in twenty-five years or so, I am alone in this house. No one to answer to, or argue with, or sort out or save or hoist or drag down the road behind me. It's weird and wonderful and probably the best thing that's ever happened to me. I can breathe. I didn't even know I wasn't breathing—that's the really funny thing.

Life can become a complete blur without you even knowing it. WE. DON'T. STOP.

My father's death was sad, but not unexpected. It was slow and tedious and terrifying. But people die. It was an amazing experience and I learned a lot about myself and the people around me.

My mother keeps spiralling into the abyss of Alzheimer's but, thankfully, she is the only one who doesn't know. Alzheimer's is a disease that hits the people who have to watch it happen much harder at first than the people who are losing themselves. You have to laugh loud and long or you won't survive it, *and* you have to lean on your friends. You have to ask for help. You can't do it alone.

And you have to stay in the moment you're in and not live even one single hour in the future. NOW. NOW. NOW.

That is Alzheimer's.

Hmmn, what else?

I'm finishing a novel, starting a new album, developing a TV series, planning tours, fixing my body, being kind to myself and putting myself out there in the universe by embracing whatever it is that awaits my participation. I'm baking and painting and walking and exercising and doing yoga and praying and thinking. And most of all, appreciating my dear-heart friends and the brilliant creative people I work with day in and day out.

But I try not to do everything at the same time.

Also, music is everything. It has revealed my own soul to me.

Mom doesn't know she's unwell. Her mind tells her over and over again that she is perfectly fine.

February 1, 2017

Alzheimer's doesn't take big things away, at least not at first. It takes very small things that don't seem all that important until you string them together. It's a disease that seems to cut the dog's tail off one inch at a time, which is just cruel and malicious if you ask me. Mom doesn't know how to make coffee anymore, or use a phone, or turn on the TV. She has no idea how long she was married, or how many kids she has or if she still has a mother or how to turn the knobs in the shower. It's all just lost. She doesn't really know how to use her blow dryer or open a can or turn on the gas stove. Alzheimer's takes away very small things.

Every single day, some part of her brain walks off into the sunset and waves goodbye. She doesn't know that she's unwell. She doesn't know that there is a dark shadow creeping through her skull wiping away important information. Her mind tells her over and over again that she is perfectly fine.

That is a blessing, for sure. The bliss that comes with her deep forgetfulness makes me truly grateful. She still knows who everybody is, she knows how to laugh and she knows how to walk down the road and eat a Dairy Queen sundae. She watches the news with me at night and always remarks that things will get better. She told me that life was upside down in the thirties, too, and that all the countries got together and fought to put things right again. That made me feel hopeful.

"Life goes on," she says to me as she colours in her book. She's presently working on a little dog walking on a rainbow. Very fitting . . .

She needs my help to put the cap back on the markers. That breaks my heart a bit.

I told Mom I was worried about the world and she told me to just live my life and help other people—that that was what it was all about. "If everybody helped everybody, the world would be perfect." Sage advice from a person who has been through a lot —a few wars, a few depressions, poverty, abuse, loss of every description. And yet, she is of good cheer. "You have to keep going no matter what," she tells me as she looks out the window at two squirrels racing up a tree. "He should spend a few hours every day watching squirrels—that would help him."

I think she's talking about Trump and that makes me kind of snort.

"You never know, Mom. That might help him."

And then she says, "Well, they must have squirrels on the planet he comes from."

She hands another marker to me so I can take the cap off.

March 18, 2017

I ask myself every single day if I am doing enough for my mom. If I am present enough and kind enough and forgiving enough and patient enough. Every night when I crawl into bed I watch the worries circle around my head like a murder of crows. There are so many of them, I can't even begin to count them all. Some of them have sharp teeth and some of them let out piercing screams. I picture my heart squeezing itself over and over again in my chest and it makes me feel so weary.

They are such random worries, so far off into the future that they are simply not worth thinking about. I keep telling myself not to live there, in a time that hasn't even happened yet, but it's hard not to. My mom lives inside each breath she draws. Never yesterday, never tomorrow, only in the breath she pulls into her tiny chest. I am trying to learn that from her.

BE WHERE YOU ARE.

When I pray, and I pray a lot, I ask for help to guide me through this maze, this labyrinth of the unknowable future, and to make me resilient and hopeful and positive and unafraid. I don't know who I am praying to. I really don't. Sometimes it just feels like I'm whispering to all the people who have come before me, calling out to them in a state of desperation.

It would be nice to pray when I don't need anything. Which reminds me . . .

My grandmother told me a story when I was a little girl, about a woman who died and went to heaven. An angel greeted her in the small white room where she had been asked to wait. The angel took her gently by the elbow and guided her towards a beautiful door covered in pearls and crystals and every imaginable kind of precious stone.

"Come with me," said the angel. "I've something to show you." And the angel opened the door. The woman gasped at the sight. The room was bigger than any room she had ever seen. Inside of it, piled thousands of feet high, were an infinite number of beautifully wrapped packages. They were of every possible shape and size, and bound beautifully with silver and gold ribbons.

"What is this place? What are all these boxes?" the woman asked earnestly.

The angel smiled and replied, "These are all the things you never asked for."

I think of that story a lot these days.

I've been terrible at asking for things, for help. I don't know why.

I always felt like to have to ask was admitting some kind of weakness.

I don't feel like that anymore.

I think we're here to help each other.

I think that is the essence of human life.

We are travelling through space and time, and we're doing it together.

How fantastic is that?

March 30, 2017

Every single day, some tiny piece of my mother evaporates into thin air. Sometimes I can actually watch it drift up over her head and spill into outer space. I suppose I could cry but I think I'm saving up all those tears for a worthwhile event. I am my father's daughter for the most part. He only cried if he really *really* had to.

A person's personality is so definite and visible, but as I am finding out, not permanent. My mom is someone else now. It's that simple. I struggle to decide whether I love her or not. My throat is squeezing shut right now.

I HATE THAT I JUST WROTE THOSE WORDS.

I would be lying if I told you that I felt love all the time. Resentment storms the walls of my heart several times a day and makes me question everything. I mean, I *love* my mom. It is a deep and ancient love that has travelled between us for all time. But at this physical place, on this earth, in this moment, I feel distant. I want the old version of her back and I can't have it. I want my guide and my mentor and my fixer and my confidante back, but she has gone away. I simply have to stop pining for something that doesn't exist anymore.

Have you ever tossed a chunk of wood into a raging river and watched it surge away? That's exactly what I am doing right now. At some point you have to let go of what was, and start building on what *is*.

We have moments where I recognize her, where I see who she was. I cherish those seconds with every fibre of my being. Her laugh and the way she walks and holds her head and shoulders. There are things that remind me of who she was and I can't tell you if glimpsing them for a moment makes it easier or harder to navigate what's happening.

Take a breath.

I have no idea what lies ahead. I have to decide things when I get up to them. I cannot plan. A plan is something that changes every few days anyway.

Compassion.

Forgiveness (for myself especially).

And repeat.

I know my mom would be really proud of me right now and that is saying something.

April 29, 2017

Still, she never ceases to amaze me. She really doesn't. Even as she walks down the dimly lit hallway called Alzheimer's, she remains ever so steadfast and determined to be herself. She fights, head held high every single day, for her dignity and her sanity and well-being. She. Is. Feisty.

She keeps us all on our toes. (I am often on my knees, but that's another story altogether.)

No, I don't know *this* new version of her very well, but having said that, I am getting to really appreciate and love the woman who is fighting to show herself to me. I have thought so much about memories, and what they mean to us as human beings—how they define us and shape us and breathe life into our humanity. What I've come to understand, through a great deal of my own anguish and heartache and sadness, is that memories DO NOT define our souls. Our souls—my mother's soul, and all the souls who are bombarded with memory loss —are intact.

I've been trying, but I can't begin to tell you what I have

learned about myself and my mom during this unfortunate but, in its way, glorious journey. I knew my mom was strong and resilient but I had no idea how strong, how resilient. She said to me once, after one of my rants where I tried to be the memory police a few years ago, that a person didn't have to remember everything in order to be happy. That, as you can imagine, kind of blew my mind for the following several weeks.

"You don't have to remember everything to be happy."

We caregivers have some kind of weird desire, or need, to remind them of what they're forgetting. To this day, I find myself correcting my mom. I want to punch myself in the throat for being an idiot. It's always about something small, but correct her I do. . . . Well, maybe not "correct," but redirect. . . .

The most important thing I have learned after the past six or seven years of losing my mother, is that I'm not losing her at all. I'm gaining—discovering if you will—parts of her I would never have known existed otherwise. In doing so, I've stumbled across pieces of myself that have made me a much better human being. My mother continues to teach me through a heavy constant mist and she lets me know in no uncertain terms that she is going to forge on and I had better follow her into battle.

Excuse me while I go get my shield. . . .

Oh wait a second, Mom says I don't need my shield. I have her.

April 29, 2017

My mom just texted me this:

"Iam well andhappyI love my catandmy lifegenemy my"

The small triumphs.

Just a few simple words.

A reminder of all the good.

Mom says you don't have to remember everything to be happy.

May 15, 2017

I don't mind crying. I think a lot of people try as hard as they can to avoid it, but I don't. I used to, but not now. I didn't like the feeling of letting myself go to that spontaneous uncontrollable place, so I tried my damnedest to contain the tears inside my skull.

I can remember how much my eyeballs ached from holding the tears back. It was a pain that seeped into my sinuses and my jaw bone and into the deepest part of my inner ear . . . but, by God, I wasn't going to unleash the waterworks. I was going to be brave and sensible and "grown up." It was a miracle that my head didn't explode.

Ironically, given my newfound appreciation of bawling my head off, I haven't really, truly cried about the death of my dad. Those tears come in little quiet bursts that disappear inside my heart like steam from a kettle. I can be standing in the shower and I'll feel my throat squeeze around my vocal cords, or I'll be in my car driving into the blaring sun and I'll feel a shard of loss pierce my temples. But I don't let it turn into anything of any consequence.

I shake my head, open and close my eyes a few times and turn up the radio.

I save my tears for little things.

Old movies and animal rescues and TV commercials about newborn babies and people who fight to save an old tree from the clutches of the government who want to build yet another road. And war and cruelty and poverty and and and . . .

I cry about the sublime beauty of art and creativity.

I cry over people who are making intricate, amazing things out of loss and pain and defeat.

I cry watching my mother colouring in her books, when I see her determined focus and her pure joy at seeing the pictures come to life.

I finally have realized that tears are worthwhile things.
They strike me as the most wonderful things on the planet.

June 21, 2017

I have a sort of constant low-grade sadness. It sits in a little
corner of my heart all the time. It's like that person we've all met
at a party, the one who seems to suck the gladness out of every
glass of champagne and every delicate piece of cake and every
colourful bouncing balloon. While I still feel grateful and serene
and optimistic, I know that the sadness will rain on my parade
if I let it. I have to be diligent about stopping it or it will be such
a downpour that the parade will be cancelled altogether.

It's okay to feel sadness. I don't mind it lingering there like
smoke. It serves as a reminder that I am able to feel things and
be present in my own life, a participant rather than an observer.
Life isn't a beer commercial. You can't run down a sunlit beach
every day. If you ask me, that would become tedious. Obstacles
and challenges simply make you stronger and smarter and
more authentic.

And my sadness is not depression. I'm not depressed, I'm sad.
Two very different things. I know why I'm sad. It isn't a mystery.
I don't want or need a pill or a drink or a salve or some sort of
magic tonic to make it go away. I am quite happy to feel sad.

My mother's illness is BIG. It takes up a lot of space in my
heart. When you lose someone you love an inch at a time, grief
hangs over every hour of your life. As my mom would say,
"That's how it goes. You've got to get on with it." So that's what
I am doing. I try not to mope and lament and wish for things to
be different. It's a waste of precious time.

My mom has never been a complainer. I've never know her
to be negative or unappreciative. She always sees the good in
everything. She gives everybody the benefit of the doubt, no

matter what they've done or how many times they've done it. She recognizes what it is to be human.

Had it not been for her complete acceptance of me, and all my shortcomings, I would never have had the courage to pursue a career in the arts. She taught me that success wasn't going to be about making money, it was going to be about making friends and connections with like-minded people.

She told me on many occasions that what I was choosing to do with my life wasn't going to be easy, but that it would be very rewarding.

And it has been that.

It's been a sublime dream.

I know beyond a shadow of a doubt that the best advice she ever gave me was to be myself. There's a song in there somewhere. . . .

July 16, 2017

My mother never speaks about dying. She only says that she plans on living a long, long time, which makes me smile, because she says the words with a seriousness reserved for heart attacks or the whispering of love poems in the dark.

"I have NO intention of going anywhere, Jann, not yet."

My father was afraid of dying. He said he was afraid of it many times in the last few years of his life. I think it was his Mormon background that made him afraid. He believed that God would surely punish him for his countless sins. He left the church as a young man—it wasn't for him, he said—and pursued a life of drinking and smoking and swearing. Things the Mormon God wouldn't think too highly of, or so he was convinced. I told him that God—Mormon or otherwise— doesn't punish people, that *people* punish people. I don't think he believed me.

My mom has always maintained an ease around death that astounds me. She has never flinched in its presence. She simply looks it in the eye and confidently says, "Not quite yet."

Even in her constant state of confusion, she remains steadfast and calm. She did tell me that she wanted a big choir at her funeral and a very ornate, very large, angel-type headstone placed on her grave.

"Well, I already got a memorial bench for you and Dad when he died, Mom. Your name is on there too. . . ." I paused because I wasn't sure I should say the next part out loud. Then I finally blurted: "If we put your name on it at the same time we had Dad's engraved, it was a LOT cheaper."

She laughed out loud. "Well, that was smart. It's ridiculous what people spend to die."

"There's an angel on there, too. I drew one and they copied it onto the marble."

"One of your nude angels?"

"Sort of."

"Marble isn't cheap."

I tried to change the subject. "I wonder where he is?"

"Your dad?"

"I think he's somewhere wonderful and interesting."

"I do too."

In the weeks after he died, as I mentioned, Mom saw him several times, usually hovering at the foot of the bed or standing in the walk-in closet. "He looked so young! Just like he did when I first met him. And he wasn't sick. He was normal."

I loved hearing her talk about those visits.

"I told him he had to go, though. It gave me the creeps."

"Um . . . yeah!"

"I told him he had to go someplace else."

"Has he come back?"

"I've never seen him again."

My mother was always matter-of-fact. She was even before the Alzheimer's. She always stated the obvious. I hope I can be more like her as I get older. I hope I can embrace the days with pure joy and a simple gratitude that transcends the real world.

I hope I can find grace.

I hope I can find peace.

I hope I can kick ass.

July 31, 2017

I'm mad at my mom so much of the time. It makes me feel ashamed and almost physically sick. I'm mad because she isn't who I want her to be. With each word my mother repeats, and every disoriented action she makes, I feel more and more twisted and discouraged.

And the guilt sets in like cement.

And my soul feels pushed into the ground.

And I doubt any goodness I may have.

I look into Mom's eyes and try to find her. This is such a shitty disease. How bound we are to our memories, and to the routines and rituals we repeat year after year after year until one day, we don't know how to do them. There are so many things I want to talk to her about, so many things I want to ask, but the days when I could ask those questions are gone. They simply get stuck at the back of my throat with the disappointment and the fear and the loss.

I try and find the good. Yes, I'm glad that she is still here with me and that she still knows who I am. She still laughs and likes to walk and have ice cream and enjoy all her darling pets. The crazy cat especially . . .

But if I'm honest, I know that the woman I love is simply gone.

I remember Mom telling me one afternoon, many years ago, that she wished Dad had had his stroke a lot sooner than he did.

"How do you figure that?" I said to her.

"Well, it knocked the 'mean' out of him. It's like being married to a complete stranger and I like it. That doesn't often happen when you've been married as long as we have."

When I laughed out loud, she wondered why I thought it was so funny. "Geez, Mom, I didn't think having a massive stroke would could have such a positive spin."

"You can put a positive spin on anything if you set your mind to it." She was so calm and sure of herself. "That's the way it is, Jann. Things happen to people in life and you just have to keep getting on with it."

"It's still scary."

"Sometimes life is scary, but you can do it."

"No, I can't."

"Yes, you can. You are."

I had to think about that one. YOU ARE.

"Nobody comes here to get it right. Boy, if I'd known how terrible your dad was going to turn out I might've run the other way down the aisle."

"You're on fire today, Mom."

"But that was my lot, and I got you kids out of it. I guess that was the point—even though you almost killed me."

"I always love that story, Mom."

"Well, you did almost kill me. But that's okay. We survived."

And we will keep doing just that.

And then some.

August 21, 2017

When someone you love has a disease, you live it with them. You suffer it with them. You hold them inside your heart, and

you breathe in what they breathe out, and you *keep on going.*
And you somehow find the grace you need to keep your head
up and your shoulders back and your hands steady.

While I walk this road with my mother I know that I am
healing myself at the very same time. As I learn what makes me
stronger, because of Alzheimer's, I realize that the path to
wisdom is rife with obstacles and I am finally embracing them
rather than running from them.

When you run from things, they run with you. Facing
adversity is the one thing that has truly made me a better, more
empathetic, interested, easygoing human being. I realize that I
learn very little from easy triumph—nothing, in fact. If
anything, easy success makes a person self-absorbed, egotistical,
selfish, bossy, entitled and pretty much devoid of kindness.

Show me someone who has struggled throughout their life
and you can pretty much be certain that you'll find generosity
in them. A gratitude that is obvious and an unmistakable, wacky
sense of humour.

Just a *good* person.

My mom tells me every day that she has a great life.

She has no past.

She has no future.

She just responds and reacts to exactly what is happening at
that moment. And the moments are good.

There is much to be gained from appreciating the exactness
of a moment. In a moment, anxiety cannot exist. You have to
fear the future in order for anxiety to do its best work.

You cannot worry about what's about to happen if you're
really and truly smack dab in the middle of the moment you're
in. Thanks, Mom.

October 23, 2017

I hadn't seen my mom for five weeks until yesterday, and it was unnerving to see the visible changes in her behaviour. When I look into her eyes, it's like there is a void that becomes wider and deeper with every passing second. She looks past me, somehow, perhaps searching for home.

She says she wants to "go home" a lot. The girls who watch over her when I am away tell her that she *is* home but my mother waves off that notion with the back of her delicate hand. She says she wants to go home even when she is sitting in her own chair in her own living room. Home is not a place, but rather a marker in time. Home is remembering who she was. Home is the absence of confusion.

I wish I could take her home but I can't. Nobody can.

My mom is in a long hallway, opening thousands of doors that reveal tiny pieces of a puzzle. She doesn't know what door she has already opened, or if she is going in the right direction. She simply keeps walking until she needs to sit down and have a cup of tea and a tart. These are her days. This is the plodding, meticulous nature of memory loss.

It's a catastrophe.

She remains cheery somehow, while I do not.

She laughs with her head back and her shoulders lifted.

I try to.

I'm trying to figure out what to do next.

We are isolated here where we live. Mom doesn't see many people, save for the girls, and the neighbours who pop in once a month or so.

I am gone a lot.

"You have to work Jann, I know that," she tells me.

To say it's hard, well, it's more than hard.

For me and my brothers mostly.

For the people who knew my mom before . . .

My mom instilled a lot of wisdom in me, so I know I'm making good decisions that she would applaud. I hear her at night telling me things when I am half asleep. She has become part ghost and part saviour and when I hear her, I am scared and relieved in one single breath.

November 12, 2017

Most days, I don't know exactly how to feel. But I don't much care about that anymore. Trying to figure out how one feels all the time can be exhausting and somewhat pointless.

Though Mom's illness makes me constantly want to evaluate my state of being. I've got one foot in the future all the time, wondering what's going to happen next. I get mad at myself for doing it.

I'm living in two very different worlds—one when I'm off working and the other when I am here in the trees with Mom. It's like riding a pendulum that swings like an old woman's breast. Well, maybe my own breast. God. Time makes fools of our bodies.

Losing weight doesn't help in that department either.

Where was I?

My mother is a lamb these days. She's quiet for the most part, always looking off somewhere I can't go. She doesn't dwell on frivolous things like clothes or her mother's china or what's happening in the world. She sits in her chair and closes her eyes and sleeps a lot of the day away. She's not agitated or worried, she's very still and slow.

When I come into the room, she glances up and says, "Oh, it's you."

"Yes, just me," I say. "Are you having a nap?"

"I think I was. Am I supposed to be somewhere?"

"Just right where you are, Mom."

"Well," she laughs. "Thank God."

She doesn't say anything about the ladies being in the house anymore. She's given up fighting for her old life. It's a blessing not to be tangled up with her every night, wanting things to be like they were. Not that she even knows what that means.

I can't remember how it used to be. I pinch my eyes closed at night in bed and try to visualize my life from two years ago, and it's just a wall of mist. I am so glad I'm busy, because if I wasn't, I think I'd spend my days crying. Not that that's a bad thing. Sometimes you gotta cry a little if you ever expect to laugh again.

November 25, 2017

I have worked so hard on myself these past two years—on my state of mind mostly. When you died, a big quiet fell over the house and the land around the house and the sky above us too. Everything was different. I felt a dull, constant drone around my body.

I kept trying to make out what the wind was saying at night. I purposely left my bedroom window open an inch or two, even when it was cold, so I could hear the trees sing. I'd lie on my back and stare up at the knots in the wooden planks of the ceiling. I thought I saw shadows that looked like people floating and it made me pull my covers up tightly around my neck. I'd finally fall asleep. Those first few weeks after your departure were a blur. And then you came by. . . .

I know you were hovering over me one night. I could feel it —I could feel you. You woke me out of a dream and pulled the breath out of my lungs. My heart sped up and beads of sweat gathered around my collarbones. I yelled into the dark and you shot up through the air like a bullet. I haven't seen you since. I think you realized you scared me.

Mom sees you all the time, still, at the foot of her bed. She says you stand there, blinking. She says you look young and that your hair is falling across your eyes like when you were a boy.

"He's not sick." That's what she says over and over about how you look when she sees you, and I'm glad that she's not afraid of you like I am.

I still get mad when I think about things you did.

I still let out a long breath when I recall the terse conversations we had time and time again. Your reluctance to show kindness and mercy.

I feel like I'm just getting to know you now that you're dead. I wonder how in the world that even makes sense.

December 10, 2017

It's ironic that I can't really remember how Mom used to be. She's been steadily changing for a decade now. The slow and tedious and determined threads of memory loss keep winding themselves around her entire body. Not just her mind.

The way she moves is different. As she walks, she swings her legs out in front of her, agitated and reluctant, as if her feet have no sense of the ground beneath them. She holds her hands together as if in constant prayer, and her head barely rotates on top of her spine as if it has been welded into two or three static positions.

It's as though her whole self is held captive by a sinister, invisible force. She looks past me somehow, as if I am beside myself and it is that other version of me that she strains to see. She squints over my shoulder and I find myself trying to step into her line of sight. I'm desperate to catch her eye.

"What are you doing, Jann?"

"What are you doing, Mom? I'm trying to figure out who you're looking at!"

"Well, I thought I was looking at you."

"You're kind of looking over my shoulder," I say as lightly as I can.

"So?"

I can't stop wanting Mom to stay in my reality. I think I've learned, but I never really do. I'm so fucking scared it takes my breath away. She's going farther away from me.

I have a hard time talking to her now, too. I mean, I talk to her, but it's very basic and repetitive and not really what I want to be saying at all. I want to beg her to come back "home" and stay with me and not leave me behind. I want to ask her a million things about what I should be doing and deciding and becoming and it's all just useless now. She can't be where I am. I don't even know if she wants to be. It's what I want, *not* what she wants.

Her contentment throws me off. She has taken her eyes off the land and pointed her soul out to sea. She tells me she is happy and lucky and that she has a wonderful life. I can somehow hear her saying, although very faintly, "You can do it. You're okay, Jann. You were always okay, and you're gonna be fine."

And then I bawl my head off.

December 12, 2017

I've wanted to write to you, Mom, for a long time. It feels like I need to do it now, before it's simply too late or too little. I've wanted to tell you so many things about growing up, and screwing up, and getting up. But I have a superstitious feeling that if I write them all down and send this letter to you, you'll disappear.

I talked to you on the phone yesterday. It's so strange hearing your voice—like it's coming through a thick wall with tiny holes punched into it. It's so familiar and yet so faded and distant, like a ghost is relaying our conversation to me from a place I can't go . . . yet.

"Everything is the same here. The cat is excited you called. She knows your voice. Do you want to say hello to the cat?"

"It's okay, Mom. I'm happy to talk to you."

"Where are you?"

"I'm in Regina doing a concert."

"Oh. Why didn't you tell me that?"

I change the subject instead of saying that I told you countless times where I am and what I'm doing. I do everything I can to *not* correct you or remind you. "Is it nice at home, Mom?"

"I don't know." You call over your shoulder to the care worker. "Is it nice here?"

You usually want to hang up. You say that you should let me go do my things and I always feel sad when I hear the click of the phone on your end.

I miss talking to you, Mom. I wonder if you miss talking to me?

I feel very alone even when I have a million people around me. I feel like I'm by myself in a room that's so deathly quiet it makes it hard to think. This kind of grief is so wide. I would rather it be a sharp point that pierced my lungs, but it's wide and dull and endless. I know you might live a long time, Mom, and I'm trying to think of what I am going to do with this distance between us.

I'm trying to get my head around how I'm going to close the gap between what is and what is not.

December 22, 2017

I stood in front of my bathroom mirror last night, after having come out of the shower. No, I did not have any clothes on. I don't usually take the time to look at myself with any kind of conscious effort, but last night I was exhausted. Even the towel in my hand seemed to weigh a thousand pounds. It was all I could do to dab the dripping water off my face and neck.

I stood there in front of my giant mirror and looked at a person I haven't spoken to much lately. She's been running around the country, trying, it seems, to keep up with a bolt of lightning, which is never easy to do.

Now I'm peering at myself. Maybe even glaring. My body has changed so much. I've lost fifty-five pounds in two years and everything has moved, gotten lower, gotten longer. Things seem to be clinging to the bone now, which I don't mind.

I actually don't mind it one bit. I don't mind all the marks that have made a map of me, the streaks that break across my stomach like they're racing to reach my belly button. I don't mind my skin, which is thinner and paler than I remember, and looks like a wet sweater hung over a chair. I don't mind the creases in my neck that weren't there before all this change. I push up all the extra stuff under my chin and smile at how silly I look, standing there, water pooling at my feet, my little dog glancing up at me from a few feet away.

"You're nude," Midi says silently. "You need to put on pyjamas and put us to bed."

Not just yet. I push my breasts up to where I think they should be and stare at the whole length of my body with intention and compassion and a whole lot of appreciation.

This body has carried me through so many adventures. This body has shown me so much loyalty.

I marvel at the sight of myself, to be honest.

I see so much beauty now. I don't know why I didn't when I was younger. I didn't see anything good, not the least bit good.

I mourn that time but can't dwell on it.

I am here now.

I have a long way to go. We have a long way to go, my body and I.

I have a feeling that I am only just now getting started.

December 26, 2017

People are afraid of change. I know that I have been riddled with that fear many times in my life. And when I felt that way, I somehow managed to rationalize that staying where I was, in a negative, unhealthy situation, was better than what lay ahead —the unknown, unpredictable future that couldn't possibly be easier to navigate than where I was. So I did nothing. I waited for my life to "fix itself," "sort itself out." I waited for time to go by, as they say. . . .

It never works.

Someone once said that change, in order to be effective, must be radical. I finally believe that to be true. Anytime I've tried to get by with small tweaks, I've always ended up by having to make giant, frightening leaps in order to alter my life path and move forward. Those damn frightening leaps . . . work.

Cutting bad people and bad situations out of your life sounds drastic and painful because it *is* drastic and painful. But it takes a long time to get to the point where you're ready to make those cuts.

Most of us know what we need to do for months, if not years, before we make a big change, but we tuck those decisions away as if we're waiting for a magical door to open. Usually by that time anything like that happens, your life is miserable, unrecognizable, in pieces.

I know because I've put off making the necessary cuts time and time again.

Fuck.

We do learn, but we learn so slowly it's laughable. We see very clearly how we're caught in these bad situations, and yet we're so paralyzed we can't break away.

Fear can fool you into thinking that you're not worthy of happiness or contentment or love. Fear takes great pleasure in keeping the human heart in limbo. It feeds on human beings stuck in a slow and constant state of decay.

I always got caught up in the details. All the "what ifs?" The details weighed me down—all those unknown factors that keep you where you are because you can't figure out a resolution.

All I can say is, if you're unhappy, make a change.

Risk it. Don't worry about the details.

The devil is in the details.

Jump, fly, leap—

Find your bliss.

December 29, 2017

I am filled with shame when it comes to my mother. She is only a hundred yards away from me in the house that she and Dad built on my property over a decade ago—*one hundred yards*. Yet I am more and more reluctant to walk over there to see her. Reluctant to stagger those measly hundred yards and sit for a cup of tea. I mean, I go over every day, but my visits are becoming shorter and shorter. I always seem to be running off to do errands or make phone calls. Or I just want to leave and go home, away from the heaviness and the heart-breaking reality of it all.

It's a grotesque feeling in my body.

It makes me anxious.

It makes me so fucking sad.

It makes me feel like my love and my affection and my ability to be compassionate towards my own mother are diminishing with each minute of each day.

This is a new stage in this dreaded disease for me. It's another rung in a ladder that constantly leads me down into the cold, hard ground. It really is a glimpse into hell.

I second-guess myself constantly. Am I doing the right things? Am I keeping Mom in her house for her or for *me*?

Is she too isolated out here where we live?

Am I being selfish? Would she be happier around more people and more activities? How long should I keep this up?

What should I do next?

I don't know.

I just don't know.

Alzheimer's is different for every person it inhabits. What it chooses to steal from each person cannot be predicted by anybody. Not a doctor on the planet really has a clue. . . .

The only thing that is for certain, is that *it will win*. That's the hardest, most hideous part of this whole entire journey: there is no hope of beating this disease.

You have to surrender to it or die trying, as my mom says now and again. "I'll die before I let this get me down." Those words ring in my ears like a bomb went off beside me. That sentence is one of the most profound things she's said to me in the past five years.

And her eyes were locked onto me when she said it. Her jaw was set, her hands were steady and her shoulders were as square as she could make them. "I'll die before I let this get me down."

It's like she was telling me what the only escape route was. It was haunting and liberating all in one breath.

No, I don't know what to do. I try and stay where I am. I try and just be with her. I fail every goddamn day—that I will tell you.

A darling friend of mine told me to read to her. "You need to read your mom your book. Reading is one of the most beautiful things you can do for another person. You really need to do that, for you and for her."

I think I'll try and do that today. I'll just keep trying.

December 31, 2017

I'm not one for resolutions. I have never made one in my entire life. Well, maybe I have, but called them something else. . . . Perhaps "commitment" is the term I've used. I've made commitments to myself, which is good, I suppose.

I have committed to saving myself. That's what I've been doing the past two years. I've been pulling myself back from a very deep, dark ocean of uncertainty. It's been hard at every turn. I have failed a lot, but within the failures lie so many intricate lessons that it's hard to reckon with them all. You have to use said lessons on an I-need-one-of-them-now" basis.

They come in quite handy. I find myself saying, "Oh yeah, I know how to do this now. I know where I went wrong the last thirty-six times, and THIS time, I actually think I know what to do."

I am a spontaneous human being. I say things and do things and immediately know whether or not that the sentence or the action is going to get me into trouble. Sometimes it is the trouble I seek, the outcome and the reaction I want to explore. It certainly keeps my life interesting. You can't be afraid of offending people, because that will happen no matter what you do.

If I am safe all the time, I'm never going to be any more of a person than I am now. And I want to be MORE. I want to stretch myself in every possible way.

My grandmother said a profound thing to me one dreary afternoon many, many years ago. "Jann," she said, "you need to spread yourself as thin as possible. You cannot expect a seed to grow when it is clumped together with a thousand other seeds. It's got to have room—a lot of room."

I'd always heard the opposite—that you couldn't spread yourself thin and expect to get anywhere.

I've never forgotten it, and I've been trying to put myself out there ever since. I don't have to be good at something in order to try it. I don't have to succeed at it, I don't have to win. I just want to do things and be as bold and as fierce as the Universe allows me to be.

Meeting new people has been my most precious thing these past few years. Finding like-minded souls who are travelling through the same mire as you. Finding that one person who makes you want to write a million songs.

Finding that kindred spirit is so spectacular. Attraction is so very rare. I know that for certain. Connection is even rarer. So when you connect with another person, put them into a jar and screw the lid on.

(Punch a few air holes though.)

Go do things.

Piss people off and ruffle feathers and rub the world the wrong way every now and again.

Get people talking.

Get people thinking.

Wake them up.

Most of them don't even know they're sleeping.

(And don't forget to poke holes in the lid of the jar.)

January 8, 2018
You are responsible for how and what you feel. It's a very hard lesson to learn. I know I've been blaming my mother for

how I feel. This treacherous avalanche that's taken us for a ride these past few years has somehow managed to bind us together like twins.

Watching my mother's illness accelerate has been like standing over a demolished, bleeding body that's been struck down by a truck full of horses (Sharron Matthews—*you* know. . . .) and watching that body writhe and twist whilst reaching a hand up begging for a tiny shred of help that you are unable to give.

Helpless.

Helpless.

Helpless.

No, life is not fair, but it is does put you through your paces.

What often looks like a disaster can lead to an explosion of wonder and goodness and an opportunity to love beyond anything you've ever experienced before. An opportunity to rise up to the very precipice of your humanity and not only survive these tragedies, but thrive inside them.

These are not bad things, they are just things. Nothing more.

Lava levels everything in its path. It isn't picky about what it destroys. It just goes where it goes. But as immediately as it annihilates, it creates. It literally makes a new world. That comforts me because I believe the same thing applies to the destruction in human lives.

When I was a kid, on the fields around us the farmers would do what they called a "controlled burn." They'd nail handmade signs on fence posts warning you of the impending smoke that would billow around our heads for what felt like days on end. The campfire smell of old dead grass and dirt being seared. I loved it, though I used to cry to Mom about all the gophers that would die, along with the mice and the ants and the other small creatures caught by the flames that marched across the fields in perfect symmetry.

"You have to get rid of the old dying stuff so the new crops will grow." That's what she'd say as she flipped her tea towel over her slender shoulder and got on with washing dishes.

I think that's what she'd be saying to me now.

I am responsible for how I feel. Not her.

And I don't just want to survive this dreaded disease with her, I want to thrive while I'm doing it.

January 14, 2018

Tomorrow, Nadine and I are going to start looking at places for Mom. I've been bawling my head off about it, but I know it's time. We are too remote out here in Rocky View County, too far removed from everything. Save for the companion care women, when I am away working, Mom is alone here. My options have narrowed and I need more help than I can provide. It sucks like hell.

Mom is changing so quickly now, and I don't want to be caught in a place where she has deteriorated to the point that it's too late to move her with any kind of grace. Nothing about this is good. Nothing about this is easy. But having said that, it's life and you have to pull yourself together and get on with it. I want Mom to keep on having a purposeful life, engaged with other people, doing activities and being surrounded with movement and motion and LIFE.

If my parents taught me anything, it was that your shoulders get broader with every challenge. They were never ones to complain or grumble about their lot in this world. They always showed gratitude and economy when it came to the shit being flung their way. It's almost laughable to think about what Mom and Dad endured in their lifetimes. My older brother's crap alone would have been enough to sink the best of us. Dad had his moments when he was far from his best self, but they always picked each other up and kept going forward, no matter what.

NO MATTER WHAT.

We had a lovely woman come out here a few days ago to help us narrow down the list of places that would be a good fit for Mom. The consultation cost $350, but I think it was worth every cent as Nadine and I would have been on a wild goose chase to find something in our general area that was suitable for Mom's needs. It's such a *Gong Show* out there. I'm finding out all kinds of things that I don't really want to know. The system is overloaded and underfunded and at a crisis point for a million reasons.

I'm scared and uncomfortable about all of this.

But I'm going to try to stay afloat for her, for my mom.

What a completely strange thing it is.

To become a new version of yourself in the blink of an eye.

January 19, 2018

I remember watching my mom and dad walking back across the yard from my house to their house one cold winter night after I'd fed them dinner. They had linked their arms together in hopes of holding each other up.

"Don't wipe out!" I hollered over the stinging wind. It was impossible to keep up with the shovelling so the path they were teetering along was pretty much made by the dogs going back and forth.

"What?" My dad turned his head to look at me and of course his hat fell off.

"Don't wipe out!"

"Jesus Christ, we won't goddamn wipe out if you stop making us lose our momentum!"

It made me laugh. I wouldn't have called what they had "momentum." My dad reached down to pick his hat up and ended up dropping the leftovers I'd sent with them into the snow. The dogs who were flanking them like a couple of enthusiastic prison guards had everything gobbled up in a matter of seconds.

Dad mumbled a string of profanities that were a work of art. The dogs looked up at him adoringly and then started barking uncontrollably, almost as if to say, "Let's get moving, people! It's cold out here and there's nothing left to eat!"

By this time I'd thrown on the pair of rubber boots that are always at the ready around my house, and sprinted out the door to help them. I didn't have a bra on so I was holding my boobs up (just to really paint a clear picture of what was happening).

"You'll catch pneumonia out here, Jann." My mom's glasses had slid most of the way down her nose and her hat had collapsed over her left eye. She looked like an ice pirate and it made me laugh even harder.

"I can't find the goddamn Tupperware." Dad was kicking the snow around trying to locate the stupid plastic container.

You have to understand that it was pitch black, minus twenty-five degrees Celsius and windy like you would not believe. We could hardly hear each other. I spotted one of the dogs with the Tupperware in her mouth, trotting merrily towards their house.

"The dog's got it!" I pointed at big white Belle, who was camouflaged brilliantly. Mom said, "Well, I was looking forward to that cake."

"It was spaghetti, Mother," my dad said matter-of-factly.

I finally managed to get everybody home and was half frozen by the time I lurched back to my place. It was a very typical night for the three of us. Just generally funny, and silly, and goddamn magical.

I thought to myself: etch this deep into the safest room in your heart and lock it away, because there won't be many more of these. I knew it at the time. I really did.

On March 1, I'm moving Mom to a new home. It's filled with sunlight and newness and good people. We are going to fix up her little room with all her favourite things. Her chair and her loveseat and . . .

God, I can't even write this. I'm crying too hard. I'm gonna stop.

You know the rest.

I can't live her life for her.

I can't save her.

I have to let her go.

I'll just love her and go up there as much as I can and keep breathing.

January 27, 2018

They say the hardest part of any journey is taking that first step. Um, it's actually the fucking packing. Full stop. Trust me.

I've been bogged down by the endless, tedious, malicious-feeling little details when it comes to my mother. All the "What about" and the "What'll I do with those?" and the ever so popular "Why the hell do they still have these?"

All the stuff . . . what will I do with all Mom and Dad's stuff?

My parents have a house full of things that are so disjointed and random and (if I may be so forthright) downright *useless*. I think my mind shut itself off about a month ago and stopped trying to deal with any of it. I simply had had enough. Between my mom and my job and my life and my own insecurities and disappointments and my countless little failures with their countless little sharp teeth that bite deep into my ego, I fell apart.

On March 1, I am moving Mom to a new home. God, I can't even write this, I am crying too hard.

I think I'm just starting to stand up now.

(I've not written a word for ten minutes while I've been staring longingly into the frost-covered trees. But I digress.)

I actually don't mind falling apart. It gives me a chance to go, "Okay, now we have something to put back together." Falling apart makes you stop at least, to look to see if you still have your arms and legs and, God forbid, your eyebrows.

Now I've made the decision. I've signed the papers. My mother would do the same thing for me, tables being turned and all that.

The tether is long between a mother and her child. It transcends physical life and the boundaries fixed by the rules of time. Breaking it would be like trying to separate smoke from itself. It is simply not doable.

Mom has had eighty-one interesting, beautiful, uniquely challenging years on the planet. If you were to ask her right now about her day, she would say, "I love my life, I love my cat and I have had a wonderful life." She says the same thing every single time.

We shouldn't judge a human life by how it ends, and we so often do. How we die has nothing to do with how we lived. I think I've been confusing these two things. I've been making her whole life about these past few years and that's not where the truth lies.

February 15, 2018

Two weeks to go before Mom moves into her new digs. It seems impossible and bizarre and a whole lot of other things. How time moves along.

How it wrinkles us.

How it shapes us.

How it pushes us like nothing else can.

I can remember when Mom and Dad were building their house here on my property. They had to live in a trailer for about ten months as construction dragged on like speeches at a wedding. My mom wanted to make the trailer "homey" so she had Dad build a makeshift deck for it out of some old two-by-fours and some tired plywood. It was rather large deck now that I think back on it, about three times the size of the trailer. My mother was *thrilled*.

They had brought a fridge with them from the old house and thought it a good idea to put it on the deck to keep extra stuff in. I mean, they more or less made themselves a "holler" down there at the end of the gravel road. If you listened hard enough, strains of banjos could be heard floating on the breeze.

The "extra stuff" was mostly beer, bags of oranges and large slabs of cheese from Costco. My dad could eat oranges like, well —I don't even know like what. Do monkeys eat lots of oranges? I digress . . .

The fridge was sitting out there in the rain and the snow and the wind and the sun. You'd think it would have shorted out, or blown up, or fallen over, but no, it stood there like a pillar of comfort and strength. When Mom and Dad ventured into town to run errands (i.e., buy more beer and cheese and oranges), they would tie their dog, Dolly, to the handle of the fridge. I could never for the life of me figure that one out. When anyone drove into the yard, Dolly would of course get up from the deck and, in doing so, pull the fridge door open. It's as if she was saying, "Here, come and enjoy a cool beverage and some snacks." It still makes me smile just thinking about it.

We've been lucky here. I've been lucky. There are so many really wonderful memories. I can taste them and feel them on my skin. They are as real now as they were all those years ago.

That bloody fridge.

That bloody goddamned fridge.

So funny.

February 16, 2018

It takes a long time to become a person. Most of us don't become a decent one for at least forty years. We are in training for decades, flailing about, leaving destruction in our wake. (Well, I certainly did. I probably still do.)

I've been trying to juggle my career, deal with the ever-changing situation with my mother, navigate my personal life (not too successfully) and just generally cope with being a human on the planet in these times. My emotions have been dangling by a flimsy rope. Low-grade depression has dogged me for a couple of years. It's there, like nausea, rising up into the back of my throat and then dropping back down into my hip bones. I am reminded of a time when I put too much laundry detergent in my new washing machine. Foam filled up the room and slithered along the hallway, down the stairs and out my front door. I kid you not. That's what this depression feels like—foam that multiplies and expands itself into the tiniest of places.

And then I wonder if it is actually depression. If I'm honest, at times it actually feels good. I know this makes no sense. But sometimes the feeling of loss and sorrow that touches my lips and strokes my hair seems almost sublime. Or maybe just like change is coming to get me.

My heart is open. It's on the outside of my rib cage and that's always a precarious spot. It can be hurt much more easily but I don't mind the risk. I would rather be hurt than not hurt. There is value in the unpleasant experiences—growth, wisdom.

My heart falls in love with all the wrong things and people, but I guess I don't mind.

It also falls in love with new songs and new opportunities and new ideas.

It falls in love with impossible things and I find that so intoxicating, considering I've been *very* sober for a couple of years.

I spent many years tucking my heart under a rug, and I don't do that anymore.

March 2, 2018

So. Life didn't stop. The world is still revolving. The sun is rising up like the sun tends to do. My mom is all moved into her new home. She is on a "memory" floor in a brand-new building in southwest Calgary, a thirty-five-minute drive from my place. It's bright and colourful and tastefully set up with soft couches and roomy chairs; lots of tables and nooks where the residents can sit and ponder and nap and dream of good days yet to come.

I was prepared for the absolute worst scenario. I pictured Mom bracing herself against the car door, refusing to get out. I had imagined piercing cries of "I WANNA GO HOME! WHAT ARE YOU DOING TO ME?! NO NO NO NO NO!"

We heard none of that. She came with us calmly and quietly and was of good cheer. She had no idea where we were.

The plan was fairly simple, but it took months of preparation. Nadine Beauchesne (and Nadine's wonderful partner, Dave) are nothing short of a miracle workers. I bet Nadine had no idea what she was getting herself into when she started working with my family three years ago. (Nadine, sorry!)

The plan was this:

Fly Mom to Palm Springs for a five-day getaway. I took Nadine and Donna Marie, one of our other main caregivers.

Nadine came back two days early and organized the main move, like the bigger items from Mom's house—her lounge chair, a single bed, a few chairs, tables, lamps, a nice area rug, paintings to hang, framed photos of family and friends, clothes, things for the mini fridge, toiletries. Everything she would need to be comfortable and familiar. Nadine had to buy a TV and get the cable hooked up. She bought two sets of sheets, towels, toilet paper. She knew Mom would really miss her animals, so she researched this robot cat, with fur, who purrs. You name it, she took care of it. She had to move Mom's life and make this new space seem like she had lived there forever. She did an amazing job.

We figured we needed to get Mom a bit disoriented, get her out of her house, so that it wouldn't feel like we were moving her out of her HOME and into a NEW WEIRD PLACE. When we landed it seemed like a good idea to go straight from the Calgary airport to the memory care centre. (That's what I'm calling it.)

When we got there, the little "Calgary apartment," which is what I told Mom it was, looked absolutely wonderful. Three hundred and seventy-five square feet of loveliness.

Mom walked into her new place and sat down in her recliner. "I recognize that picture." She pointed at a painting hanging on the wall in front of her. She's had it for fifty years.

Everywhere there were little bits of her life and her mind seemed to accept it as familiar and warm and real. She was everything I thought she wasn't going to be. She liked it. She liked the cat. She was serene and easygoing.

Though she was disoriented, for sure, and eventually we all had to leave, except of course for the staff who were buzzing around making Mom feel welcome and introducing themselves.

It was weird.

It's still super weird.

Normal? Well, normal is an ever-changing thing.

The real pets are a bit scrambled. Belle seems down. She stays with Midi and me, and I hope she will adjust eventually. She is getting extra treats and extra walks down the road. She's at my feet as I write this, sighing every few seconds if I don't talk to her.

Last night she sat on Mom's front step and howled. It was heartbreaking. She'd howled on and off throughout the day. I walked her through Mom's house twice, just to show her that no one was there. It gave me a lump in my throat the size of a horse. She reluctantly came with me. She slept here for the first time last night and did pretty well. I got up a few times to talk to her and let her out to pee.

The cat has gone to live with Donna Marie. They are good pals and I know he's going to have a great life. It was hard splitting up Belle and Lucky, but such is life. When I travel, Belle will go live with Nadine and Dave as she loves them and knows them. We all have to make adjustments and get on with these new versions of our lives.

I am headed to see Mom in a few hours.

Nadine saw her yesterday and Mom told her that she had lived there about a year! We both are gobsmacked at how she has taken to all of this. I know these are early days, but so far, she is cheerful, chatting with people, sitting in the common area and walking around, eating well, being friendly. I could not ask for more.

I feel relieved, sad, happy, up, down. You name it.

This is not only a new chapter, but a whole new book.

March 18, 2018

Mom has been in her new "home" for just about two weeks. I've been away for pretty much that entire time. I had a massive press junket for the new music to motor through, which kind of sucked (the timing, *not* the junket—for that, I am overflowing with gratitude), but the show must go on as they say in the theatre. Mom would want me to be working and doing and being and living as large as possible. She has always been my biggest cheerleader.

I know it's only been a couple of weeks, but I swear when I saw her she looked smaller to me, if that's even possible. Alzheimer's seems to shrink people like good cashmere sweaters in a hot dryer.

Also, the bridge that makes up four of her front teeth is getting fixed so it wasn't in her head. People look so strange without their teeth. It aged her thirty years, her cheeks were so sunken. She keeps asking me where her teeth are and I just kept answering, "They're almost fixed, Mom. You'll have them back in your head soon! Nadine took them to the dentist and he's almost got them ready to go."

"She took my teeth to the dentist!" she exclaimed. "I look like an old lady!"

"You look great, Mom."

"You think so?"

"You always look excellent."

"Well, you look pretty good too." And then we laughed until it got quiet again. The silence seemed long to me. The kind of silence that makes space itself push out into nothingness. I broke it by offering her a piece of flaky, syrupy baklava.

"That looks delicious!" she said as she reached for it. "Did you make that, Jann?"

I *love* that she knows my name and that she Still. Knows. Me. I hope she doesn't forget me. I hope her brain hangs on to my face for as long as it can.

"I did *not* make this. I can't really bake, Mom."

"Well, you used to be able to bake. You baked for me when I was a little girl."

That pretty much cracked every rib in my body. I felt them snap one by one as my heart expanded into a small version of a burning sun.

"You baked like mad," she said.

I thought back to a time not so long ago where I would have corrected her. How selfish I was, how naive, how blind. My desire for her to get things right, to beat Alzheimer's at its own wretched game, trumped kindness and compassion and patience.

I was afraid. And I thought I could change what was happening.

"Well, I'm glad you and Dad liked my baking back in the day," I said. "I'm glad I didn't kill you with raw cookie dough."

"SO AM I!!"

We laughed again and then walked down the well-lit hallway to her room and her robot cats. Yes, she had more than one now—after the staff saw my mom with her cat, the manor bought two more and soon Mom had all of them with her. She thinks they're hers.

"I was crying all day waiting for you to come," she said as we sauntered arm in arm.

"Why were you crying?"

"I was crying?" she said, her head cocked to the side. She had bits of baklava stuck to her lip.

So goes the wheel. Spinning like our tiny blue planet through the cosmos.

March 31, 2018

It's been a month since we moved Mom into the care centre. (I can't bring myself to call it a nursing home.) I walked over to her house today and it feels completely bizarre. Like there was a death. In a way, I guess there was. Someone had left the radio on, tuned to the CBC. When I walked in the door and heard voices, it startled me.

There was a split second where I thought Mom would be sitting there eating some kind of cake and drinking cranberry juice. She loves cranberry juice. I hate it. There were boxes still on the floor, filled with odds and ends, and mucky footprints trailed around the kitchen island. It's like no one ever lived there. There are just ghosts now, and piles of books and magazines, and cupboards filled with china—dozens of delicate cups that have no saucers. I don't know what I'm going to do with it all. I can't think about it right now. I can't decide one more thing.

I walked over here to see if Mom had a can of coconut milk, which she did, and I ended up sitting on her couch, staring out the window at the birds picking away at the old, dry sunflowers. I looked around at everything and pictured Dad in his chair, feet up, eating mini Oh Henry bars. I can't tell you if it made me feel profoundly sad or the tiniest bit serene. Maybe somewhere between the two . . .

Souls take up so much space. They are big and all-consuming. They are tangible physical presences that you can feel. What I thought about mostly as I sat there in Mom and Dad's empty house was that they were both fine. Dad is still Dad, even though he's somewhere else entirely. Our bodies wear out, and we basically move out and move on. I love thinking about that. I am not afraid of it at all.

Mom's soul is standing guard over her tired-out body. She is "beside" herself waiting to step into another realm, another version of her journey. Her memories are intact somewhere, her essence and her personality—all of it—waiting for her. Even if you can't believe that, it's a beautiful idea. If you can, it's a comfort.

I walked back to my place with a bag filled with more stuff that I don't need. An old mechanical bear that my granddad had for years. I know my little brother wanted it. He looked lonesome sitting on the shelf, so he came along with the coconut milk and a tea cup with images of Prince Charles and Diana. I actually found the saucer.

Oh life, what a crazy damn ride.

May 6, 2018

It's hard to write about my mom these days. Even when I am sitting right beside her, she's a million miles away. She looks past me like I am made of smoke and beams of light. I honestly don't feel sad anymore. Sometimes giving in isn't a bad thing. It isn't a weakness or a failing or a cop-out but, rather, a giant leap of faith.

My mom does not know where she is.

She does not know who she is or what she's done in her life.

She doesn't worry about dying any more than she worries about living. She is in a state of NOW.

It's constant and pounding and insistent and it doesn't give two giant craps about the future.

There is no future.

There is something very graceful about not knowing.

She does not seem to feel afraid or have a single worry. If even a hint of anxiety enters my mom's body, she forgets it immediately. These states can't exist in her because she can't hang on to them. Trust me when I tell you that there are a few times every day when I envy her.

My life sometimes goes too fast for me and with the speed comes uncertainty and doubt and a fair bit of self-loathing.

I do my best not to look around and compare myself to other people, but that can be impossible. Even when I think I'm not, I am.

It's interesting to me because I know better.

I have confidence, but very little self-esteem, and believe me, the two can co-exist.

Most of the time, I manage to keep the heaviness safely tucked away. My mom was an incredibly strong and resilient woman. She gave me all the tools I need to navigate this crazy life, and what she ran out of time to teach, I know I can figure out myself. I have good friends and they are at the centre of all my joy.

But I miss my mom.

I'm glad she still remembers a little piece of me.

May 15, 2018

I don't know where I begin and end some days. I have become someone who adheres to a simple yet strict routine, so as to maintain my crumbs of sanity and my ever-fragile sense of well-being. I know I am not the first human being on the planet to lose her parents. I'm not foolish enough to think that I am the only one wandering the earth orphaned and alone. But that's how it feels.

Our parents die, and all of us go through a metamorphosis of sorts. That change moves into our every breath and forces us to stand on our own two feet. We're orphans.

My mother is still alive, but it doesn't feel that way. She feels gone.

She has forgotten her own life. She has forgotten who she was and I doubt very much she has any idea who she is now. It bothers me in ways that will take me years, if not the rest of my life, to come to terms with. Perhaps it's because my brothers and I are merely ghosts to her now. We are these entities that float through our mother's mind like whispers of long-lost words and photographs that make no sense to her at all. I want to stand on the top of a hill and scream things at God that would have the angels lock me away.

Now, more often than you might think—when I'm running the vacuum over the kitchen floor or folding laundry or brushing my teeth—tears push themselves out of my eyes without warning. So much for saying I'm not sad anymore. They physically hurt my face. They hurt my jaw and my teeth and my hair. I stand as the vacuum whirs and the water runs in the bathroom sink and the warm tea towels fall idly onto the counter and I cry as quietly as I can. I wonder where my life went. I wonder when I'll feel normal again.

Is it possible that I feel *embarrassed* that my own mother has forgotten me?

It seems like the ultimate insult to an otherwise good and comfortable relationship. Mom and I came so far only to have Alzheimer's happen.

I'm at a time in my life where it would have been so nice to ask *her* about her life and her politics and her sensuality and her ethics and her dreams. My younger self never thought about those things much. My younger self only saw me in the mirror and didn't so much as notice my mother's brilliance and intelligence and strength. We always seemed to talk about me and what I was doing, and not what my mother was doing. I wonder now what difficult things she endured in order to protect me. What's lost is lost. She herself would tell me to let it all go. I'm trying to.

But I waited too long to ask her the important things. The grief is awe-inspiring. It's bigger than any relationship I've ever messed up or lover I've lost or defeat I've experienced. This is the greatest loss of my life, losing her while she stands right in front of me, wondering who I am.

May 22, 2018

There is no piece of my life that remains unchanged. It's as if a magician (or a maniac) fanned out a deck of cards, asked me to choose one, and then without any hesitation simply threw the rest up into the air, head back like a Pez dispenser, and started laughing. A big machine-gun laugh that shot out of his mouth, ripping the air in half.

The magician is life.

The card in my hand is me.

I still have me. I chose me.

I miss my mom when I am in a room with her, and that feeling is magnified when I am three thousand miles away in London, England. I have tried to FaceTime every day or so, with Nadine operating things on the other end. Mom is perpetually cheery and smiling, and more often than not pushing a red velvet cupcake into her head. Off camera, I can hear Nadine telling me that they "hit the coffee shop, hence the cupcake" and we all laugh.

"What did we hit the coffee shop with?" Mom says as she flashes her newly minted smile. (She hasn't lost her new teeth, praise the Lord.)

"Jann knows we went to the coffee place."

"How does she know that?"

"She can see your cupcake." Nadine brushes some crumbs off Mom's lap.

"I'm gonna get fat." Mom empties her lungs with another big laugh.

I tell her that's what she's supposed to be doing. My mom couldn't be fat if she tried. I, sadly, took after my dad's side of the family. Shall we say, sturdy? Yes, they were sturdy folk, hearty, steadfast. I have vivid memories of my dad's mother eating bread and butter over the kitchen sink. She was a big woman who passed away too early of complications from diabetes.

Not that I need another reason to keep looking after myself.
I haven't had a drink for two years.

Best thing I ever did.

I don't know why it took me so long to figure out that
sobriety is the best drug. Everything takes its own time, I
suppose. Things happen when they happen. I come from a long
line of bad drinkers so it's not hard to understand what I was up
against. I just thought I was exempt, somehow, from the weight
of history and genetics. I wasn't.

I'm home tomorrow, and have spent the last few days
catching up with dear friends here. Nigel, my English
gentleman, has gone through pretty much the exact same thing
as me the past few years. His father had dementia and passed
away last year. He's presently emptying his parents' house,
which for at least a hundred years has always had a member of
his family living in it. I don't feel so bad!

He's sending me home with a ceramic bedpan that, he tells
me, "every member of my family has shat in." Okay, I know
that's gross, but we really laughed.

May 25, 2018

Something very small made me realize that I have become a
decent, responsible, caring human being.

Birds singing.

I always knew they were there, off in the trees, talking to
each other, but I don't think I really listened to them. When I
came to the simple realization that I really cared about their
delicate songs, that I cared about the living things around me,
I felt a huge sense of relief. I think *all* of our problems come
from not caring about other people, animals, trees, the Earth in
general. Indifference and complacency have isolated us from
each other.

Children *always* appreciate the bees and butterflies and cats and dogs and flowers and trees and water—they see these things and they marvel at them all. Their little bodies understand the worth and the weight of what makes them feel good.

Then something happens where all those things disappear from view. We drift away from those delicate, intricate, "small" things that literally ground us and keep us content and calm and whole.

I remember the day when I saw everything again. I was mowing the lawn and I went past one of my father's rain barrels. The ever-present barrels that he had at the end of every eavestrough, collecting water for the plants. As I went past one of the barrels, I noticed a moth flailing around in the water, drowning. I stopped the mower, and walked over and scooped her out and set her on a rock where the sun was shining. I know it seems trivial, but it was such a moment for me—I felt so good. Not a lot of things were making me feel good at that time, but that small gesture made me feel that I was going to be able to go forward in my life with renewed purpose and meaning.

It kind of blew my heart into a thousand pieces, actually. I started paying attention to all the tiny things that had been trying to rescue me. The birds singing and the leaves rustling and the wind blowing my hair into the side of my mouth. There was a definite hum everywhere. I don't know how I'd tuned it out for so long. I guess I was running in the wrong direction. I was running away from who I was. Perhaps this all seems trite, but to me it's been a revelation.

Stop long enough to hear birds singing some time.

The sound will find its way into your broken heart, the one you didn't even realize wasn't working the way it should.

June 10, 2018

When I went to see my mother yesterday, I found her in the dining area with her new friends. She was having some soup and laughing about something one of the other ladies had said. She saw Midi first, and lit up, and then she saw me.

"Well, for God's sake," she said, as she always does. "It's you!"

"Yeah, it's me!"

She turned to her pals and introduced me with an enthusiasm that was utterly heartwarming.

"This is my mom!" she said, pointing at me. I didn't correct her. I just smiled and gave her a kiss.

"You're my mom too."

She thought really hard about that. "I am?"

"Yes, you're my mom too."

"Well, that's hard to believe!"

She seemed filled with the joy of a new discovery. It resonated with me like some kind of song. I marvelled at how happy she was over something so simple.

It's so easy to lose sight of what makes us happy. What gives us serenity and satisfaction and an overall sense of well-being. We all just want to feel secure and comfortable.

It doesn't matter how much money you have or what dream job you've got or how other people perceive your life. *Things* don't matter. Stuff is just that, temporary and disposable. But the way your brain works and how that delicate balance of chemicals makes you *feel* is pretty much everything.

I am learning from my mother that I have to keep moving. That my life is not static and that sadness and anxiety and worry and doubt are not static, either. They change and morph into glad things and easy things and happy things just as easily as they can turn even darker. Emotions are kind of like the weather, always changing. Storms can't last forever. Optimism is mighty.

Mom once told me that the best thing about Alzheimer's is that you forget to be afraid. I will never forget those words for as long as I live. At least I don't think I will.

We all seem to live so far into the future, planning and configuring and sorting and filling our calendars, that we forget where we are and who we are. I don't live in the future. My mother has taught me to be where I am. I'm happier. I'm more content. I feel a sense of ease I didn't have two years ago, when I was so worried about things that hadn't even happened yet.

Small things.

Small.

Bring huge victories.

June 14, 2018

The world is in trouble, not that it hasn't been before, but we need to look at ourselves and really start basing our decision-making not on the promises that politicians make, but on their character. On who they are, how they live their lives, what they believe to be ethical and fair and gallant.

Progress comes from the efforts of many like-minded people, who want to see good things come to life: effective economics, rational development of our cities and towns and industry and agriculture and natural resources. It does matter *who* is making the promises, not just what those promises are.

Voting has never been more important than it is now. Participate in your world. Choose good humans to lead us and let's help them make our country better. These good and ethical people might not be in the party that you've historically supported—maybe they're an independent or someone on the other side of the aisle.

I really try to find out who my representatives are as people. What they stand for, beyond partisan politics. We all need to take a little bit of time to find out more about the people who want to represent us and not merely cast our votes to the abyss. Just think about what our neighbours to the south are dealing with now.

June 26, 2018

I don't know if I even have the courage to write these words down. I've been thinking about what they would look like on a page for days, weeks even. I wondered what the consonants and the vowels would feel like as I tapped them into being. I wondered what would happen to my soul after I breathed them to life. Would I go to hell?

I guess I'll find out.

I went to see Mom on Sunday. She was still in bed when I got there around two in the afternoon. She didn't feel good. She kept repeating, "I'm so sick, Jann. I'm so sick. I don't think I'm going to live."

I kept asking her where she felt sick and she said, "Everywhere."

"Your tummy?"

"No—everywhere."

"Does it hurt?"

"No. I just feel sick."

I sat on the bed beside her and folded my fingers into her fingers and told her she wasn't going to die.

"Okay," she said.

"Okay," I said quietly back.

She looked right at me then and it shook me somehow, like I had mistakenly bitten into a piece of tinfoil.

The words *I don't know who you are* shot through my brain, and they scared me. I felt ashamed. Where did that come from? It was as if they had been lying just beneath my skin and they finally jabbed their way out, and it hurt.

My own mother, lying there staring up at me, saying my name like she had a billion times. I drew in a breath and felt my entire childhood fly through my torso in a split second. I wanted to cry but nothing came out. I just held on to her hand, this person whom I had always loved so fiercely.

I don't really know what I'm writing down.

I don't know what I'm trying to say.

I am appalled at my failure to remain loyal and steadfast.

My memory is failing me too.

I can't remember her.

I frantically sift through the files scattered in my head and I cannot picture her—the mother I always knew.

I hope she comes back. She used to be safe in there, but my image of her is waning and I am so fucking afraid.

August 11, 2018

I haven't written for a while. I've started a few times and then just set it aside to putter around the house or spend time in the yard or walk the dogs.

My mom has unbelievably entered her sixth month at the "manor." We moved her at the end of February and, honestly, it seems like it could have been yesterday, never mind half a damn year ago.

These days I am surrounded by an eerie calm. I feel like a tornado came through the yard and wiped any remnants of my parents' lives away and now it's quiet and motionless. The eye of the storm.

Their house sits a hundred yards across from me and I look over at it constantly. I don't want to, but it intrudes like a giant tombstone. Nadine and Donna Marie have all but cleared it out. I wasn't much help. It made me profoundly sad. All the things people gather around them—eighty years of things that only mean something to their owners. The rest of us stand with our hands on our hips and wonder, "What the hell was this for? Why would anybody need this many of anything?"

My mother's prized possessions: china figurines and ceramic collector's plates with scenes of kittens or ducklings in baskets, dozens of teacups, countless lamps and chairs and rugs and frying pans and plastic wrap by the mile. Hundreds of framed pictures and so many clothes . . .

It simply overwhelmed me.

It's jarring and profoundly difficult to go through a person's life possessions. It feels voyeuristic and very wrong. Like prying into a person's secrets and then, after finding said secrets, simply giving them away. Actually, if I'm honest, throwing them away. My parents had an edition of *The Joy of Sex* under a bunch of magazines in their closet, which made me smile and shudder all at the same time.

I didn't want to find anything that changed my idea of them. And then it dawned on me that perhaps I didn't really know them at all and that made me swallow hard.

Who were they?

They're gone. Which means I can't really find out now.

I know my mother is alive in body, but the person that I knew is gone. I visit someone who feels like a very distant relative or a neighbour who lived around the corner from us a hundred years ago. She speaks mostly gibberish—sentences that have no origin, no topic, no connection to anything. They are just words she says and those words are almost always followed by the most beautiful laugh.

She always tells me she loves her life, and I am completely bowled over by her earnestness.

"I want to live as long as I can!" she insists.

If that doesn't tell you something about the human spirit, I don't know what will.

[CONCLUSION]

Final words. Well, nothing is ever final, but here goes.

There are so many layers to all of this. Every day presents new and unseen challenges when it comes to dementia and Alzheimer's. I have said this many times before, but it all feels to me like the old adage of cutting a dog's tail off one inch at a time. It's horribly uncomfortable and impossible to anticipate or measure. Even the doctors will tell you that they don't know how fast it will go—that there's no way to tell because it's different for every patient. And on and on it goes. I left many medical appointments about my mom feeling completely defeated because I hadn't learned one new thing. Despite the doctor's level of compassion, I felt alone.

I remember one visit where the doctor said to me, "We won't actually know that your mother had Alzheimer's until we do a postmortem."

I was like, *What? What do you mean? Like when she's dead? That's when you'll know what she had?*

After that, what she had somehow didn't seem as important anymore. I just wanted my mom to not be scared. I wanted her to be comfortable and safe and engaged and entertained. You don't have to remember what you did five minutes ago in order to have a good time. Vodka taught me that. (Thank God, that lesson regarding vodka is one I've unlearned, though it sure applies to being with my mom.)

155

And the story of living with this disease is different for every family. I just hope that by sharing this diary, I have hit on some helpful notes for you and the people you love and care for. I think the one thing that resonates with all of us who are going through this is the helplessness you feel, the anger and the frustration and the *fear*.

I kept telling myself early on that I couldn't do it.

I can't.

I just can't.

I'm scared.

I'm so goddamn ready to knock your block off. (Meaning, yes, my mother's block.)

Why are you doing this to me?

I feel like my life is falling apart!

I was so busy being mad that I forgot about love.

And yes, you can forget the love you have for the person who is going through this heartbreaking disease. As they disappear, inch by inch, the love you feel has a big fat question mark at the end of it. "Do I know who this person is?" "This isn't who I used to know." "I feel like they've become a complete stranger." "They don't know me anymore."

But you do know them. And you know you *love* them.

I believe with all my heart that love permeates Alzheimer's. It gets through even though you think it's not getting through. It's like a shard of light that even a blind person can see. Love will surprise you at every turn. You'll discover parts of your heart that you never even knew existed.

I am a better version of myself because of all of this. Looking after her has been—and is—an honour. I continue to learn and grow, and I know for certain that I am getting braver.

—

Good things come out of bad things. It is one definition of our humanity—to face such difficult times with grace and compassion and to help another human being get through the tough bits. That's what life is all about. My greatest successes have nothing to do with my music career. They have nothing to do with awards or accolades or money. My greatest successes are my friendships, the weight and authenticity of my word, and my ability to stretch myself into the far corners of sadness and grief and loss and be okay with being there, because it's just life being life and it's temporary.

You have to decide that you're going to go where they go, though, or you really, truly, will be left behind. It's the best thing I ever did. I gave in, let go, succumbed, surrendered— whatever you want to call it. You need to stop correcting them, and just love them and follow them into the fog.

It's a revelation, I will tell you that. Alzheimer's is going to win, so you have to become a beautiful loser! That sounds ludicrous, but it's so damn true. I thought I could force my mom into remembering everything and all I did was alienate myself from her life. Agreeing with her and accompanying her on her journey changed me. It really did.

My mom spent almost a year in a memory care facility in Calgary, Alberta, about thirty-five minutes from her old house, which still sits across the yard from mine—a lonesome reminder of another life and another time. Some days it strikes me like a giant tombstone, and other days it's like a beautiful church. I can almost hear songs pouring out of the windows and I can almost smell Dad's peanut butter cookies baking— that glorious scent wafting across the garden. The birds are still warbling and Mom's peony plants are falling onto the greenest grass on the planet. It's like they are still there. I cling to memories, as we all do. They make me who I am.

Mom had visitors every day. Donna Marie Dillman and Ginny Smale, two of the "homeless women" who looked after her for years, still went to see her and helped me with her care. Nadine Beauchesne orchestrated Mom's appointments and made sure her daily routine was watched carefully. I visited three or four times a week, though I was busier than ever. I was able to be a daughter. I wasn't scared anymore. I wasn't mad. I was on an adventure with Mom. She was a mighty tree and I got to be one of her myriad branches. It was such an honour.

She liked it there, in her new place. She told me that every time I saw her.

"I have nothing to complain about," she'd say. And after that, I admit, would come a lot of gibberish. Disjointed sentences and sentence fragments. She had slowed down so much. Her spine looked like the arch of an old church and she seemed to have delicate new lines on her face and hands with each passing week: a map perhaps of every place she'd ever been.

I would ask her if she was scared of dying and she'd reply with the sureness of a judge handing out a verdict: "No! Why in the world would I be scared of dying—it's the easiest thing in the world."

Have you noticed that I'm talking about Mom in the past tense?

In the middle of December 2018, she rapidly started to decline. A few weeks earlier, she had been diagnosed with a urinary tract infection so bad she had to be taken by ambulance to emergency. Through some miracle, I had the day off from my lengthy tour and was able to fly into Calgary to be with her. She was obviously very confused when I got there, hooked up to the heart monitor, people coming and going with a manic purpose—bright lights and bells and buzzers sounding off somewhere every few seconds. Hospitals were never one of Mom's favourite places to be—are they for anybody? Nope.

Not surprisingly she was of very good cheer, laughing that indelible laugh of hers. Throughout her stay, she was kind and helpful and polite to every nurse and every doctor and every attendant that poked her or flipped her over or took her blood pressure or lord knows what else. She was always brimming with positivity. That was Mom. "I have a good life," she would say every single time you visited her.

But after that hospitalization, she never quite got back to where she'd been. When she returned to the memory care "manor," her head hung down in the most uncomfortable looking position, and she wasn't able to swallow any more. She *forgot* how to swallow. That is a textbook Alzheimer's progression. It had to have been scary and frustrating for her, although she never let on or expressed any kind of anxiety or fear. She was always calm and steadfast.

She went as far as she could go and then I think made the decision to just get going.

She became completely disinterested in eating, "pocketing" food into the side of her cheeks, or wrapping it in a napkin and tossing it, or shoving it into a plant. She didn't want to eat simply because it had become such a difficult thing to navigate. Try as they might, the staff slowly began to realize that it wasn't something that was going to improve.

I had made plans to spend Christmas with some friends in England. When I got on the plane, I pretty much knew things weren't looking good. I was supposed to fly home on December 29. Two days before the return flight, Nadine called me and told me that Mom was very lethargic and not wanting to get out of bed. I remember saying, "Nadine, I know she's going to die.

I need to call my little brother and I need to get home." Pat was working the oil patch in northern Saskatchewan and needed to arrange a flight.

The manor's policy is to call an ambulance when a client is in medical distress, but Nadine let me know when it arrived and I refused to let the paramedics take her to the hospital. I didn't see any point in giving her an IV drip of fluids and antibiotics, hooking her up to a heart monitor, and dragging the whole horrible thing out even longer than it had already gone on.

I don't understand our culture when it comes to end of life. We make sure our beloved pets don't suffer, but often drag our dear humans through one useless intervention after another, causing who knows how much pain. Our whole approach to dying needs to be reimagined, revamped and retooled.

Thankfully, Pat was able to get a flight to be with her, and I made it home six hours before she peacefully passed away.

She knew we'd made it.

She knew we were there.

She never forgot us. She knew who we were, she knew our names and she knew we belonged to her. I'm so grateful for that.

Nadine was there, too, and Pat's wife, Jodi, and my dear friend Janine Violini was there as well. She's worked with me for ten years, and then trained to become a very gifted death "doula." She was able to explain what was happening to Mom as she made her way out of the world. The information, the enlightenment was a game changer. It brought so much clarity and order and calm and comfort.

After my dad died, I regretted not having spent time with his body, or engaging in any kind of ritual or ceremony. We all simply gathered up our things, pulled the sheet over his head and left in a fog of doubt and grief.

With Mom, Janine took us through a lovely journey of

saying goodbye, which began with showing respect and admiration to Mom's body, which had carried her so courageously through her life. It had worked so hard and been so faithful to Mom. We surrounded her with fresh flowers, washed her face and hands and feet with lavender water and put cream on her hands and feet, telling her all along how much we loved her.

Then Janine cleansed her energy and we helped wave her spirit out through an open window. It felt beautiful and healing.

Alzheimer's was no foe for my mother.

Somehow, she managed to maintain her positivity and show me that she was in there from time to time. Even in her death, she gifted me with so much grace.

I know she's free. I know she's on to another adventure, one I am not able to join her on as of yet. I know she is restored.

I asked Mom many years ago what she'd like me do when she died. "What would you like mom? Like, you need to tell me because I don't have a clue . . ."

She thought about it for what seemed to be a very long time. Then finally she said, "Well, I don't care what you do with my body, honestly, do whatever you think. But I wouldn't mind a big choir."

So . . . I got her a big choir.

What a journey this has been. What a goddamned, wild and wonderful journey this has been. I made a lot of mistakes but I did some things right, too.

All you can do is your best. And also don't forget about love. Mom never did. So make sure you love as hard as you can.

Mom always told me, "The best is yet to come. . . ."

And I believe her.

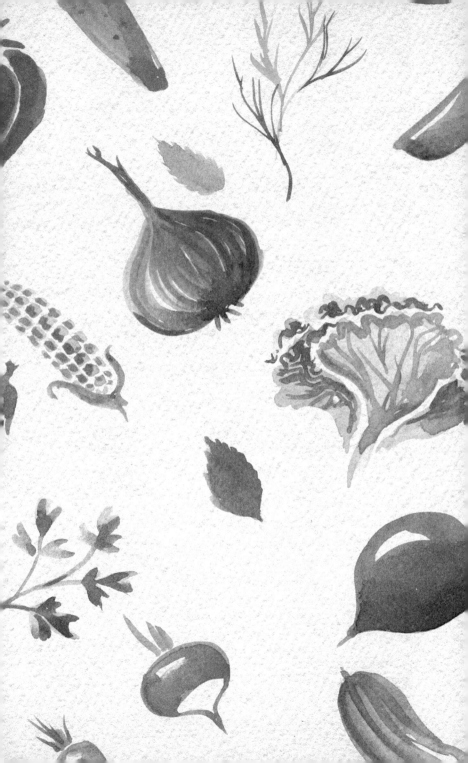

What I Fed My Mom (and My Dad, Too)

Food—eating it, preparing it, planning it, talking about it—
became a major theme in the care plan with both my parents.
My dad was always concerned with what he was going to eat
next, obsessed actually, and my mother could not have cared
less. It was hard getting her to eat at all. It was tricky keeping
them both interested and organized when it came to meals, so I
basically needed to teach myself how to cook nutritious,
interesting, *easy* lunches and dinners. NO pressure!

I'm laughing now, but there was about a year when I felt like
I was sinking, especially when it came to suddenly having Mom
and Dad at my house for most of their meals. I felt frustrated
and angry for about six months because I didn't know where my
own life began and ended. Then very magically one day (or so it
seemed) the three of us found a rhythm. I began to feel the joy
that comes when you help somebody else, when you give of
your time and your heart. And imagine my surprise when I
realized how much simply feeding people played into their
health and harmony and my peace of mind.

I was very conscious of time, and how much of it I had every
day to devote to figuring out how to keep them happy, because
at the end of the day, their well-being was my number one
priority. They really looked forward to the meals I prepared.
Mom always came over all dressed up, with earrings and nice

shoes. It kind of broke my heart to see her treating the short walk from her house to my house as a big outing. I thought I would only be cooking the occasional meal to help them out, but it turned into feeding them the majority of their meals for four years.

When you sit at a table with family and friends, you talk. You look at each other, you ask questions and hear stories. I will never regret the hundreds of meals I shared with Mom and Dad and the countless things I learned about their lives. I really got to know them on a level that I am just now fully understanding.

Of course, there were times when I literally threw things together that I had in my refrigerator or in the pantry, and there were other times when I tried to make special things, not only for them, but for myself. I am not a chef. I'm not trained in anything culinary nor do I possess much skill with a knife, nor do I know any of the terminology that a true foodie would know like the back of their hand. But I do love food and feel a true curiosity about life in general, and that's what inspired these recipes. I wanted to feed the people I loved *good, simple, easy food*.

Everything I've included here I made time and time again; they are recipes that both my parents loved to the point where even my mom would ask for seconds.

I hope you enjoy making a few of them for your loved ones. They really are dummy-proof and I am proof of that! Add your own touches and don't be afraid to modify them any way you want. The basic map is there and the rest is up to you. I think I fed my dad about nine hundred pizzas towards the end of his life, he loved them so much. He could eat two pizzas all on his own and he never stopped telling me how good they were. That will always be a beautiful memory for me.

I wish you lots of love on your own special journeys with your dear hearts.

Eat, drink, and be of good cheer. It's only life being life and you can handle much more than you think.

PS: Eat dessert first whenever possible. (Mom told me to tell you that.)
PPS: She also said, "A little piece of pie never killed anybody."

GUILT-FREE FLOURLESS BANANA-PEANUT-BUTTER-EGG PANCAKES WITH MAPLE SYRUP

2 eggs

1 banana

¼ cup peanut butter, or almond or cashew butter

pinch salt

I love to eat these at least once a week!!

Put all the ingredients into a blender and pulse until well mixed. It'll look like pancake batter, only a little thinner as it has NO flour.

Set a frying pan over medium heat and spray it well with nonstick spray, or they will stick. Pour the batter into small dollar-sized pancakes and cook for 30 or 40 seconds a side. (Don't make them very big or you won't be able to flip them. #truth)

This recipe usually makes about 20 pancakes. I smother them with butter and maple syrup. So did Mom.

WATERMELON, RED ONION, FETA AND MINT SALAD WITH LIME AND HONEY DRESSING

4 cups roughly chopped watermelon, well chilled

1 medium red onion, thinly sliced

1 cup crumbled feta cheese

1 cup torn mint leaves

DRESSING:

juice of 1 lime

2 tbsp honey

2 tbsp white wine vinegar or apple cider vinegar

pinch salt

Get a large bowl and throw in your chopped watermelon, sliced onion, mint and feta. Toss gently, so as to not mush up your watermelon. Set aside.

I use a jar with a lid to shake up my dressing, but you could also mix it in a small bowl. Juice your lime, add your honey and vinegar and pinch of salt, and mix or shake well. Pour over your salad and be sure to coat everything as evenly as possible—you don't need very much dressing. Even though it doesn't look like a lot, it's plenty!

Serve it straight away—this salad can't sit for very long, as it starts to wilt immediately.

FENNEL, GREEN ONION AND RADISH SLAW WITH CREAMY, SPICY PEANUT DRESSING

3 large fennel bulbs, trimmed and thinly sliced (Save a few fronds for garnish.)

10–15 radishes, thinly sliced

2–3 green onions, sliced into small pieces

¼ cup chopped peanuts (I like salted ones)

DRESSING:

¼ cup peanut butter

¼ cup rice vinegar, or to taste

1 tbsp fish sauce

½ tsp salt

½ tsp cayenne

½ tsp sesame oil

I use the common round red radishes, but you can use any type of radish you have on hand. I have used a mandolin and I've used my food processor and I've done it by hand with a sharp knife—slice the fennel and radishes any way you choose, just don't chop your darn fingers off.

To make the dressing, put everything in a small bowl and mix very well. It takes some elbow grease for sure. It's very thick to start off with, but loosens up as you get going. Set aside, then give it another quick mix before you pour the whole works over your salad.

Take your sliced fennel, radish and green onion, and put them in a large bowl. Mix them up with your fingers. Toss with the dressing.

Chop up some of the fennel fronds you've saved and sprinkle over each serving of salad. Add some crushed peanuts on each dish as well—as little or as much as you like.

CARAMELIZED ONION AND BLUE CHEESE PUFF PASTRY TART

1 pkg puff pastry, thawed

¼ cup olive oil

2 tbsp butter

2 white onions, thinly sliced (mild Spanish work the best)

2 cups sliced mushrooms— whatever you have on hand; use a variety if you like

½ cup sliced, pitted Kalamata olives

½ tsp salt

½ tsp pepper

pinch cayenne

1 cup grated Parmesan cheese

¼ cup crumbled blue cheese

3 tbsp balsamic vinegar

This makes great finger food when you cut it up in little hunks. Puff pastry is in the frozen food section of your grocery store. Do not buy phyllo pastry—it's an entirely different thing.

Make sure your puff pastry is completely thawed before you roll it out into a large rectangle that's about 10 by 14 inches. Don't worry what it looks like! Rustic is good—just make sure it's not thicker than ¼ inch. Line a cookie sheet with parchment paper and place your rolled-out pastry on it. Set it aside.

Set a deep-sided frying pan over medium heat and add the olive oil and butter. Add the onions, mushrooms and olives, get them cooking down and then add salt, pepper and cayenne. Sauté everything for 6 or 7 minutes, stirring constantly because it burns easily. Add the balsamic vinegar, stir well and cook for another minute or so. Remove from the heat and set aside to cool for 10 minutes.

Preheat your oven to 375°F. Poke the dough with a fork 6 or 7 times—this will keep it from bubbling up too much. Spread half of the Parmesan cheese on the dough, then the cooled mushroom, olive and onion mixture on top of that. Sprinkle with the rest of the Parmesan cheese and the blue cheese, spreading evenly.

Pop the tart into the oven for 35 minutes, or until golden brown. I can always tell by the sides of the dough how it's going—they should be a fairly dark golden brown colour.

Let cool for 10 minutes and then slice into squares.

FRESH MOZZARELLA, GARLIC, OLIVE OIL AND SEA SALT ON TOASTED BAGUETTE

1 baguette, sliced into ½-inch slices on a slight angle

2 garlic cloves, peeled and left whole

sea salt

olive oil

fresh mozzarella

These are so darn good—you'll eat 3 or 4 before your guests even get to your front door.

Brush your slices of baguette lightly with olive oil and set them on a baking sheet.

Toast them under the broiler in your oven until evenly toasted. Keep your eye on them—it doesn't take long! I'm telling you this because I've burned them dozens of times! Do not do anything else. Watch the damn oven.

Remove the toasted baguette from the oven and immediately rub your garlic over each piece of baguette. I usually go through two whole cloves.

Rip the fresh mozzarella into chunks and put them on the toasts. You'll want them to look pretty uniform. Drizzle more of the olive oil over each piece and sprinkle with some sea salt.

CHEESE AND ONION HERB BREAD

½ cup milk

½ cup water

2 tbsp butter

2 cups all-purpose flour

1 tsp fast-rising yeast

1 tsp sugar

1 tsp salt

1 egg

1 cup grated cheese (You can do two or three kinds to make up the cup if you want.)

2 green onions, finely chopped

A handful of chopped fresh herbs. Dill and thyme work really well.

Super easy. You can throw in any herb you love. Best of all, you don't have to be a baker to make this stuff.

Set a saucepan over medium heat. Add the milk, water and butter, and heat until the butter melts; set aside.

In a giant bowl, combine one cup of the flour with the yeast, sugar and salt. Stir the dry stuff together really well.

Crack the egg into the dry mixture, break it up with a fork and stir it around for a few seconds. Now add all your milk-water-butter mixture. Roll your sleeves up and start kneading everything together IN the bowl, adding the cheese, green onions, the herbs and some more of the flour. You want to make a nice ball—NOT too hard, NOT too much flour. You may not use the entire other cup of flour . . . I usually don't.

You don't have to take it out of the bowl, which is why I like this recipe —it's NOT messy. Keep kneading the dough in the bowl for a few minutes and make a nice ball. Set aside at room temperature for about an hour or so (you can cover the top of the bowl with a tea towel if you like). Preheat your oven to 350°F.

Transfer your dough into a well-greased and floured cake or loaf pan depending on whether you'd like a round or a rectangle loaf, or whatever you've got on hand. I have even done little separate buns in a muffin tin. I usually cut a cross into the top of the dough with a sharp knife, which makes it rise a little better in my opinion.

Bake for 50 minutes, or 22–25 minutes if you're doing the muffin version. Keep an eye on the bread, and remove when slightly browned.

FOUR-BEAN VEGETABLE "STEWP"

¼ cup coconut oil or olive oil

1 medium onion, roughly chopped

1 medium red pepper, finely chopped

1 carrot, finely chopped

1 cup green beans, trimmed

1 garlic clove, crushed

1 tsp mild curry powder

1 tsp cumin

2 tsp salt

1 tsp pepper

1 tbsp apple cider vinegar, or to taste

1 19 oz (540 mL) can black beans, rinsed and drained

1 19 oz (540 mL) can kidney beans, rinsed and drained

1 19 oz (540 mL) can pinto beans, rinsed and drained

1 19 oz (540 mL) can stewed tomatoes, with their juice

2 tbsp ketchup

4 cups (1 L) water

You can use any beans that you want here—just drain and rinse them well. Don't use lentils—it's not the flavour we're going for in this recipe. It's a great stew to freeze—often I'll double it so I have extra.

Set a large, deep-sided frying pan over medium heat. Add coconut oil and all your chopped veggies, garlic, spices, salt and pepper, and stir them together well. Splash in your vinegar and sauté for at least 5 minutes, or until your onions are translucent. Add the tomatoes with their juices along with the beans, ketchup and water.

Simmer it all for 45 minutes. (This recipe is also great in a slow cooker —throw everything in and set it on low for 6 hours.) I usually make it in the morning and leave it on low for a few hours.

Serve with a chunk of the herb bread, or any crusty loaf, to sop up all those great flavours.

SPLIT PEA SOUP

¼ cup olive oil

1 smoked ham hock (ask your butcher)

1 large white onion, chopped

1 tsp cinnamon

1 tsp garam masala

¼ tsp cayenne pepper

salt and pepper, to taste

2 cups split green peas, rinsed well

8 cups (2 L) chicken stock

You can completely do this vegan too—screw the ham hock and use veggie stock and a few splashes of liquid smoke. If you don't have stock, you can just use water (though if you're using the water it tastes better if you have the ham hock).

Set a soup pot over medium heat. Drizzle in the olive oil, toss in the ham hock and onion. Add cinnamon, garam masala, cayenne, salt and pepper. (I use about a teaspoon and a half of salt to start but end up adding more to taste before I serve it.) Sauté the onion and the ham hock, getting a good sear on the ham, cooking until the onion is softened. This usually takes me 7 or 8 minutes. Add the stock and an equal amount of water—about 4 litres of liquid in total.

You're going to simmer this stuff for at least 2 hours. When the ham is falling off the bone, take the entire thing out of the pot and cut all the meat off into little pieces. Chuck the bone in the garbage and put all the chunks of ham back into the pot with your rinsed peas.

Simmer for another 45 minutes until peas are soft.

You're just about done.

At this point I take a hand blender and blitz it in the pot 5 or 6 times to break some of the peas into a paste, which naturally thickens the soup. You can also take about a cup of the soup and pulse it in a blender and then pour it back in the pot if you don't have a small hand blender.

Taste your soup.

You may need a bit more salt, you may need a bit more cayenne, you may even need a bit more cinnamon—taste it! Easier to add than take away. Making things too salty sucks.

PULLED CHICKEN NOODLE SOUP

1 heaping tsp coconut oil or olive oil

1 medium onion, diced

3 medium carrots, diced

3 celery stalks, diced

3 or more garlic cloves, peeled and sliced (I use an entire bulb but I don't want to ruin your relationship)

1 tbsp salt, or to taste

1 tsp ground black pepper

¼ tsp cayenne

¼ tsp cinnamon

2 cups chopped cooked chicken (I like using some white and some dark meat.)

12 cups (3 litres) water or chicken stock

a handful of fresh parsley

2 green onions, finely chopped

½ cup small dry pasta—small shells, alphabet or broken spaghetti

Any kind of chicken you want to use will work—barbecued, grilled, baked, boiled, a rotisserie chicken from wherever—whatever you have. Coconut oil is supposed to help with memory so I used that stuff on everything for Mom—I even "buttered" her toast with it.

Put the coconut oil in a soup pot over medium heat. Add your onion, carrots, celery, garlic, salt, pepper, cayenne and cinnamon. Cook for a few minutes to soften your veggies, then add the chicken. I like using some dark and white meat. I usually cook this mixture together for 5 or 6 minutes to get some caramelization going.

Add your water or stock and simmer for 30 minutes. Add the dry pasta and simmer another 10 minutes, or until the pasta is cooked. Add the green onion and parsley and season with more salt and pepper if it needs it.

TURKEY CHILI

3 tbsp olive oil

1 onion, chopped

1 lb ground turkey or veggie crumbles

3 tbsp chili powder

1 tsp cumin

salt, to taste

1 19 oz (540 mL) can diced tomatoes, with their juice

1 19 oz (540 mL) can kidney beans, rinsed and drained

1 19 oz (540 mL) can black beans, rinsed and drained

¼ cup ketchup

2 tbsp balsamic vinegar

1 tsp sugar

This recipe can totally be vegetarian—just swap the turkey for veggie crumbles, which you'll find in the produce section of your grocery store. It's great on its own or over rice, pasta or baked potato.

Set a large, deep-sided frying pan over medium heat. Add the oil, onions and turkey (or veggie crumbles) and get it all browning. Add the chili powder, cumin and salt and stir well to coat everything.

When your turkey and onions are cooked through, add the tomatoes and beans, ketchup, vinegar and sugar. Simmer for 30 minutes. If you like, serve with a dollop of sour cream or a handful of shredded cheddar. Dad liked both.

AHI TUNA WITH ROASTED GARLIC CHIPS AND HOISIN HOT SAUCE

¼ cup hoisin sauce

2 tbsp hot sauce

1 tsp sesame oil

2 tbsp coconut oil

8 garlic cloves, sliced as thinly as possible without cutting your fingers off

1 8 oz filet sushi grade tuna (I'm warning you, it's expensive, but sometimes just what you need.)

salt and pepper

In a small bowl, stir together your hoisin, hot sauce and sesame oil. Set aside.

You'll want to put a frying pan big enough to fit the entire piece of tuna over high heat. Add the coconut oil and your thinly sliced garlic. WATCH IT LIKE A HAWK. It will brown almost instantly. As soon as it's golden, get it out of the pan and onto a paper towel.

Season your tuna steak with salt and pepper and put it into the pan. This, too, will cook very quickly. You don't really want to do anything but SEAR the steak—no more than 90 seconds a side. Remove from heat and let it rest for a few minutes. Now slice the tuna into bite-sized pieces. Spoon on some of your hoisin mixture and top with a few garlic chips. Serve at room temp with some stir-fried veggies in winter, or salads like the two on the previous pages.

TURKEY MEATLOAF WITH ZUCCHINI AND CARROTS

1 lb ground turkey

1 egg

1 small zucchini, grated

1 small white onion, diced

1 carrot, grated

1 garlic clove, minced

¼ cup ketchup

2 tbsp sriracha

2 tbsp olive oil

2 tbsp soy sauce

1 tbsp Worcestershire sauce

salt and pepper

½ cup bread crumbs (You can use ground flax instead, but it's got a very distinct taste so beware—I love it, but some people hate it.)

The great thing about this recipe is that you can put everything into one large bowl . . . and it's got tons of veggies that people won't even know they're eating.

Preheat the oven to 375°F.

Get an 8x4-inch loaf pan ready, greased and floured, or use parchment paper like I always do.

Roll up your sleeves. In a large bowl, get mixing with your hands and, in my case, wrists. Incorporate everything together and then transfer your "meat ball" into your loaf pan and stick it into the oven for 50 minutes.

Some people make a glaze out of equal parts ketchup and corn syrup, but honestly I would rather just eat it on its own. Mom liked having this recipe with a can of beans and some tomato slices. It was never too fancy around our house.

CHICKEN PARM
(THAT ANYBODY CAN MAKE)

4 boneless, skinless chicken breasts

1 cup panko or dry bread crumbs (I have even used crumbled corn flakes in a pinch)

1 tsp cayenne

1 tsp salt

1 tsp pepper

1 tsp oregano

1 tsp garlic salt

2 eggs

1 cup shredded mozzarella

½ cup grated Parmesan

1 jar of your favourite spaghetti sauce (Honestly, who has the time?)

Preheat your oven to 425°F.

Put each individual breast into a resealable bag. I use a rolling pin to pound the breasts down into a flatter version of themselves. Put the panko in a large bowl with ALL the spices. Mix well.

Beat the eggs in a separate bowl big enough to dip the chicken breasts into without making a complete mess. Dip each piece, shake off the excess egg, then dip into the panko and cover them completely. Set them on a sheet pan covered with some parchment paper . . . you HAVE to have some parchment, otherwise it's a nightmare to clean!

Put the chicken in the oven for 18 to 20 minutes. Remove the chicken at that point and cover each breast with a dollop of tomato sauce (from a jar of your favourite spaghetti sauce) and a big handful of the mozzarella and Parmesan. Put them back into the oven for 5 to 6 minutes. (Then I like to put them under the broiler for 60 seconds at the end to get the cheese kind of burned. Well, not quite . . . you don't have to do this last step, unless you love that almost crispy and golden cheese as much as I do.)

FOOLPROOF "TESTED A THOUSAND TIMES" PIZZA DOUGH

2 tsp fast-rising yeast (or one packet, if that's what you've got on hand)

1½ tsp sugar

1 generous cup very warm water

¼ cup olive oil

3 cups all-purpose flour

1 tsp salt

I used to do this by hand, but now I use my KitchenAid with the dough hook. Doing it by hand works just as well, but needs elbow grease and some patience.

Combine your yeast, sugar, warm water and olive oil in a large measuring cup. Stir gently and set aside. Put your flour and salt into a large mixing bowl and stir well.

When your yeast has activated (a few bubbles on the surface), add it gradually to your flour as you mix it on a slow setting. Make sure it's not too wet—you want the flour mixture to be able to form a ball and NOT stick to the sides. Same goes if you're mixing by hand. Add a little more flour if you need to.

Then I leave my mixer on knead for 7 or 8 minutes. Remove the dough and set on a well-floured surface. Shape the dough into a ball and knead a few more times. (Or knead by hand on a well-floured surface until the dough feels springy.) Cover with a clean tea towel and leave it for an hour to rise.

Preheat your oven to 450°F.

After it's risen, roll it out, put it on your pan, cover it with a little tomato sauce and your favourite toppings, and bake for 15 minutes.

Extra!

You can also use this dough to make naan bread. Pull off a small ball of dough. Roll it as thin as you can and fry it in a hot frying pan. I use spray oil directly on the piece of dough and I sprinkle it with a bit of salt. Flip it when you see the dough bubble up—it will only take a minute on each side, if that.

SHRIMP OR FISH TACOS
WITH ASIAN SLAW

SHRIMP:

25 or 30 peeled and deveined raw shrimp

3 tbsp soy sauce

3 tbsp sweet chili sauce

1 tsp sesame oil

2 garlic cloves, crushed

SLAW:

1 pkg shredded coleslaw mix

a handful of cilantro (Some people hate cilantro and if you're one of them use parsley or even basil.)

3 green onions, chopped

¼ cup salted peanuts

1 red pepper, thinly sliced

1 carrot, shredded (I like extra carrot; usually the pre-made slaw mix has some in there.)

DRESSING:

¼ cup olive oil

¼ cup rice wine vinegar

¼ cup soy sauce

splash of sesame oil

juice of 1 lime

½ tsp salt

½ tsp pepper

pinch cayenne

1 pkg corn tortillas

This seems like a lot of steps, but it's super easy to do. Honestly, I don't have the time to chop the cabbage for the slaw—I want fast and easy!

Put the shrimp in a bowl with all the marinade ingredients and refrigerate for at least an hour.

Put all your slaw ingredients into a big bowl. Mix or shake the dressing ingredients together and pour it over the slaw. You'll need lots of room to mix in the dressing—it can be messy! Put it in the fridge to chill.

Set a frying pan over medium heat. Throw in your shrimp, marinade and all, and cook until the shrimp are a solid pink colour.

Take out your tortillas and heat them up in the oven for a few minutes, or in a frying pan like I do—a little nonstick spray does the trick for easy flipping. Take 3 or 4 shrimp and put them in your tortilla, top with some slaw, fold and eat. Simple and good . . .

EASY VERMICELLI BOWL

1 pkg vermicelli noodles, thick or thin, entirely up to you and what you can find at your grocery store

2 tbsp coconut oil

1 bunch broccolini or broccoli, cut into 1-inch pieces

2 celery stalks, cut into chunks

15–20 snow peas

1 red pepper, cut into 1-inch pieces

4 green onions, cut into 1-inch pieces

2 tbsp soy sauce

1 tsp sesame oil

salt and pepper

chili flakes or hot sauce (optional)

TOPPING:

½ cup peanuts, chopped

2–3 green onions, chopped

1 tbsp rice wine vinegar

This is something Mom really liked me to whip together on nights when we got home late from seeing Dad. It's vegan, too. . . .

Soak your noodles in hot water as per package instructions. They usually need 7 or 8 minutes to soften up.

Get a wok or large saucepan going over high heat. Add your coconut oil and ALL the veggies. Add the soy sauce and stir constantly for 3–4 minutes. You want them to be crunchy—not soft and without colour.

Add your sesame oil for the last minute, along with a little salt and pepper, and I personally like some chili flakes or hot sauce.

Drain the noodles and get yourself a bowl. Serve the noodles with the veggies on top with a handful of crunchy peanuts and some green onion. The very last thing I do is sprinkle it with some rice wine vinegar—I love the bite it provides.

MAPLE AND GINGER SALMON
WITH GREEN ONION

½ cup maple syrup (use the real stuff for crying out loud)

1 thumb-sized nub of fresh ginger, finely grated

½ tsp cayenne

1 tbsp coconut oil

4 3-oz salmon filets

salt and pepper

2 green onions, finely chopped

This is a good one to scale up or down, depending on how many you have coming for dinner. And again, it's so easy.

Preheat oven to 425°F.

In a bowl, mix together the maple syrup, ginger and cayenne. Set aside.

Set a big oven-proof skillet on the burner on medium high. Heat up the coconut oil in it. Sprinkle the filets with salt and pepper and lay them skin side down in the hot pan. DON'T FLIP THEM! Cook them for 2 to 3 minutes.

Remove from heat and pour over the maple syrup mixture. Bake in the oven for 10 minutes, until the glaze is slightly caramelized. Sprinkle with green onions and serve with white rice or a side salad.

BLUE CHEESE AND
ALMOND ASPARAGUS

1 big bunch asparagus
(15–20 spears)

3 tbsp butter

¾ cup crumbled blue cheese

¼ cup slivered almonds

salt and pepper

A great side dish with pretty much any protein or pasta.

Blanch the asparagus until fork tender. I prefer them a little more on the firm side. Remove from water and set in a shallow casserole dish. Immediately cover with butter, blue cheese and almonds, and salt and pepper to taste.

ROASTED ONE-POT WHOLE CHICKEN DINNER WITH SPUDS AND PEAS AND CARROTS AND ONIONS

1 large white onion (or whatever onion you happen to have on hand)

2 large carrots

2 potatoes

¼ cup olive oil (plus more as needed)

salt and pepper

pinch cayenne

1 roasting chicken (they are usually between 3 and 4 pounds)

2 tbsp seasoning salt (your fave)

3 whole garlic bulbs (yes, I mean the whole thing, not 3 cloves)

1 cup frozen peas (or fresh, if you have them)

This could not be more straightforward.

Preheat your oven to 425°F.

Cut up the carrots, onions and potatoes into medium-sized chunks. Put half of them in the bottom of the pot. Drizzle with olive oil, sprinkle with salt, pepper and cayenne. Plunk the chicken on top of the veggies. (I rinse the chicken and pat it dry because that's what Mom always did.)

Smother the bird with olive oil and rub in your seasoning salt and some pepper.

Stuff the rest of your veggies around the chicken, including the garlic with the tops of the bulbs cut off with a sharp knife. Don't slice your fingers off as I have done several times.

The pot I use belonged to my mom's mom—it's an oval ceramic pot that is stuffed to the hilt by the time I have everything in there. I can hardly get the lid on, so don't worry if you think your pot is too full.

Drizzle some more olive oil on the veggies and add a bit more salt, pepper and cayenne. Cover and put it in the oven for 45 minutes.

Don't worry about it, it's fine.

At the 45-minute mark, take the lid off and try not to burn the hair off your arms. I have done that a million times and I never seem to learn, but perhaps you will heed my warning. . . .

Put the chicken back in the oven for 20 minutes. You can tell a chicken is cooked by looking at the legs (drumsticks)—if the skin has split away from the joint to the rest of the body, you're in good shape. Throw in the peas in the last ten minutes. Your other veggies will be a little charred and broken down but that's perfect! You can take a fork and pull at the flesh of the leg to make sure it pulls away easily.

Do not take the chicken out of the pot. Take the whole pot out of the oven and let it sit for 10 minutes and then cut it up IN the pot and get all the juices and the veggies mixed up in everything. It should just fall apart. You don't have to do anything fancy with carving this thing, just cut or pull it into pieces, then dish it up with some of that roasted garlic and the juices and veggies and call it dinner.

Save the carcass for soup. I throw the whole thing in a resealable bag and use it later in the week.

ROASTED GARLIC AND PARMESAN TOASTED BREADCRUMB SPAGHETTI

2 slices whole grain bread (or whatever you have kicking around)

1 box thin pasta—spaghetti, vermicelli, spaghettini—all work

¼ cup extra-virgin olive oil

8–12 garlic cloves (so yes, the whole bulb if you're brave like me and Mom), chopped

salt and pepper

½ tsp chili flakes

1½ cups freshly grated Parmesan cheese (Asiago works too)

a few sprigs of chopped fresh parsley

It sounds a bit complicated but it's super-fast and super-simple and damn garlicky and good.

Turn the bread into nice medium-sized crumbs. I find a food processor the easiest way to do it, though a blender works in a pinch.

Boil a pot of water—4 or 5 litres for sure. Salt it very well and add a glug of olive oil. Some people say you shouldn't do this, but I find the oil makes the pasta easy to deal with after you drain the water. While the pasta is cooking (9 or 10 minutes, until al dente), heat the olive oil on medium heat in a large saucepan. (I use a wok.)

Add your chopped garlic. I like to see the chunks, so don't chop it too finely. Once it's in the oil, stir constantly. It will brown very quickly. DO NOT BURN THE GARLIC! Add salt and pepper and chili flakes, stir stir stir. . . . Now throw in the bread crumbs. Stir stir stir. . . . After you've stirred it for 4 or 5 minutes, you'll notice it toasting to a beautiful golden brown, which is exactly what you want. Set aside about a half cup of the crumb mixture to sprinkle on top of the pasta right before you serve.

Drain your pasta, reserving ½ cup of the water. Set it aside. Add the pasta directly to your saucepan (or wok) and stir in the garlic mixture. Then add your pasta water a bit at a time to loosen things up slightly and create a bit of a sauce. You don't want it watery, so be mindful to keep it on the thick, pasty side. Add the Parmesan cheese and stir to incorporate it evenly.

When you plate the pasta, add some more cheese, fresh parsley and a bit of the garlic-crumb combo you set aside. I also like to drizzle a little bit of olive oil on top of everything at the end too. Heaven.

CHEDDAR, ONION AND
MUSHROOM QUICHE

2 tbsp butter

½ cup white onion, diced

1 cup mushrooms, sliced

salt and pepper

5 eggs

¼ cup half-and-half or whipping cream. (Don't use milk here as it makes the quiche too watery.)

1 green onion, chopped

1 cup shredded cheddar cheese, or cheese of your choice—they will ALL work fine

1 frozen pie crust

Preheat your oven to 350°F.

Set a frying pan over medium heat. Add the butter. Add the onions and mushrooms and salt and pepper to taste, and cook until soft.

In a large mixing bowl, beat all 5 eggs and cream with a fork until thoroughly combined. Add the cooked onions and mushrooms, green onion and half the cheese to the eggs and fold in well.

Lay the crust in the pie plate and poke it with a fork to keep it from puffing. Pour in the egg mixture and sprinkle the remaining cheese on top. Bake on the middle rack of the oven for 35 minutes.

EASY FOUR-CHEESE MAC

2 cups dry macaroni pasta

2 tbsp butter

2 tbsp flour

1 ½ cups milk

salt and pepper

½ tsp cayenne

½ cup panko crumbs

1 cup shredded old cheddar

½ cup crumbled blue cheese

½ cup grated Parmesan cheese

½ cup grated Swiss cheese

Preheat the oven to 375°F. Cook your pasta, drain and set aside.

In a saucepan, melt butter over medium heat. Add flour to make a paste, stirring constantly to keep it from burning. Whisk in your milk and bring it to a simmer, stirring until it bubbles and thickens. Add all your cheeses, salt and pepper and cayenne and make sure everything is melted and stirred together.

Put your cooked pasta into a casserole dish, pour the cheese sauce over the pasta and stir together. Sprinkle the panko crumbs evenly over the top. Bake for 15 minutes, let cool for 15 minutes and serve.

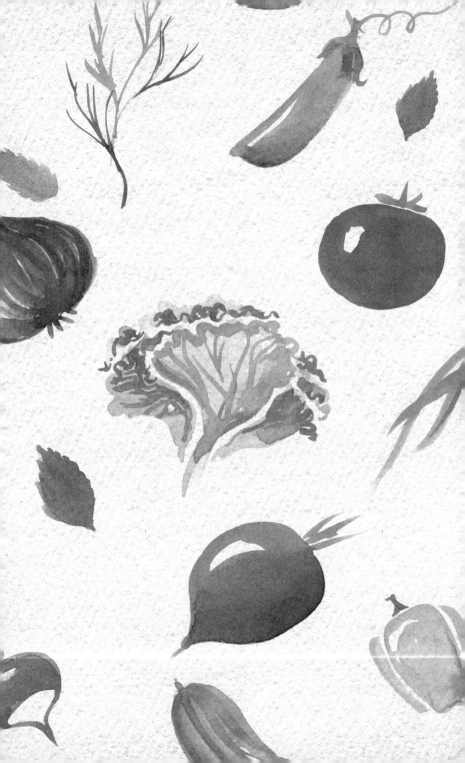

[ACKNOWLEDGEMENTS]

Thank You

I am so grateful to the amazing group of caregivers who looked after Mom with me seven days a week, pretty much twenty-four hours a day. We relied on, and still cannot live without, your humour, grace and patience, your kindness and generosity of spirit. Without you, my brothers, Pat and Duray, and I wouldn't have been able to manage. A heartfelt thank you to Ginny Smale, Donna Marie Dillman, Donna Godlonton, Montana Hancocks, Sheila Silla and Jenna Cameron.

I also want to thank Theresa deWaal, Laurel Frezell, Bev Oldham, Lisa Almond, Pat Hillcof and Sherry Lewis, my wonderful women friends who have helped me out whenever something came up over the last few years—when I had to travel unexpectedly or was in some other kind of a bind. These fine souls showed up with food in hand and smiles on their faces! Speaking of food, thanks to my old friend and cooking pro Julie Van Rosendaal for making sure that somebody else besides me could follow my recipes.

And, lastly, I would be completely lost without my friend and fearless leader, Nadine (Deneen, as Mom calls her) Beauchesne. She manages to keep us keeping on with determination and impeccable organizational skills. Nadine, you always go above and beyond to make sure Mom is having loads of fun and that she is safe and well.

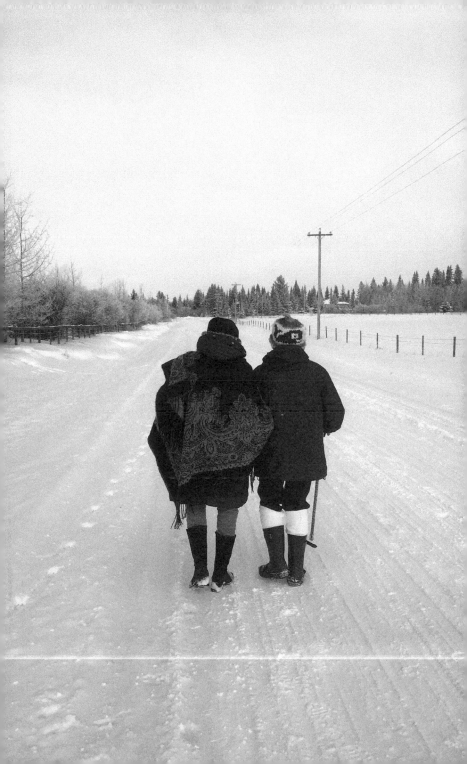

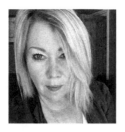

JANN ARDEN is a singer, songwriter, broadcaster, actor, author and social media star. The celebrated multi-platinum, award-winning artist catapulted onto the music scene in 1993 with her debut album, *Time for Mercy*, featuring the hit single "I Would Die for You." A year later she had her international break-out hit, "Insensitive." She has written three previous books, including the #1 bestselling memoir *Falling Backwards*. Her book *Feeding My Mother*, first published in a different edition in the fall of 2017, was an instant bestseller. She is much in demand as a public speaker, a favourite frequent guest on CBC's *Rick Mercer Report* and a guest host on CTV's *The Social*. Find her on Twitter @jannarden, on Facebook and on Instagram.